BADASS PREPPER'S HANDBOOK

T0120186

BADASS PREPPER'S HANDBOOK

Everything You Need to Know to Prepare Yourself
for the Worst

JAMES HENRY

Skyhorse Publishing

Skyhorse Publishing books may be purchased in bulk at special discounts for sales promotion, corporate gifts, fund-raising, or educational purposes. Special editions can also be created to specifications. For details, contact the Special Sales Department, Skyhorse Publishing, 307 West 36th Street, 11th Floor, New York, NY 10018 or info@skyhorsepublishing.com.

www.skyhorsepublishing.com

10 9 8 7 6 5 4 3 2

Library of Congress Cataloging-in-Publication Data is available on file.

Cover design by Rain Saukas

Print ISBN: 978-1-62914-732-1
Ebook ISBN: 978-1-62914-863-2

Printed in the United States of America

TABLE OF CONTENTS

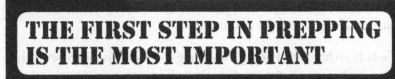

THE FIRST STEP IN PREPPING IS THE MOST IMPORTANT

The single most important step to prepping is to simply start doing it. This may seem easier said than done if you are on a tight budget, but it's the truth. The most important and difficult thing for people to do is to just get started doing something.

Many people tend to feel so overwhelmed with the huge list of things that should be done to prepare for a doomsday event that they never 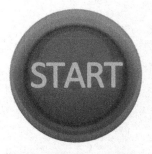 actually take any steps to get started. Looking at prepping like this is backwards thinking. It's extremely important that you break prepping down to its individual components and tackle them one by one. Remember that old saying that says the way to eat an elephant is one bite at a time? This is especially true when it comes to prepping.

Even the preppers with the most impressive stockpiles and plans started somewhere. Do you know where they started? They all started at the beginning, just like you will. It's true that some people have more money and resources than others, but everyone started somewhere.

There are plenty of wealthy individuals who haven't spent a single cent prepping despite the fact that they have unlimited resources. Likewise, there are plenty of people who barely get by from month-to-month who have a rather impressive stockpile of supplies and well-thought-out and designed emergency preparedness plans.

As you are reading through this book, try to keep things in perspective. You may end up choosing to adopt some of the advice that is given in this book and ignore other parts of it altogether. Remember that prepping is a process and it's one that most preppers never actually complete. We're constantly prepping and doing the things that we think will help us survive doomsday.

The bottom line is that doing something to prepare is much better than doing nothing at all. Some of you will choose to only do a few things that are outlined in this book. Others will go to the extreme end of the spectrum and do much more. The important thing is that you do something—and the goal of this book is to help you do just that!

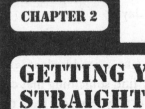

CHAPTER 2

GETTING YOUR PRIORITIES STRAIGHT FROM THE BEGINNING

One thing that all good preppers have in common is that they have their priorities straight. They have all come to a point in their lives that has enabled them to make a real commitment to prepping. It's one thing to say that you would like to start prepping, but it's something entirely different to actually make a serious commitment to start and stick with it.

If you really want to be a prepper, you need to make a commitment to prepping. If you're on a budget, this will likely mean that you'll have to make some personal sacrifices. You'll need to take a close look at how you spend your money and find ways to free up money to buy prepping supplies.

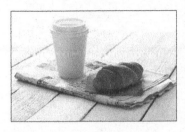

Now, before you say that there's just no money in your budget to start prepping, you really should challenge yourself to take a good, close look at your budget and do an "honest" evaluation. You may need to be brutally honest with yourself and ask some tough questions.

For example, if you think that it's impossible to start your day without stopping by your favorite coffee shop for a grande low-fat latte with a double shot of espresso, you're probably not being honest with yourself.

These are the types of things that people can cut out of their budget to free up money that can be spent on prepping. Let's take a closer look at this example. If you spend $3 a day for your gourmet coffee, that's $1,080 that you're spending each year just to feed your morning coffee habit. This doesn't even include how much you spend in gas to make a special trip to the coffee shop every day!

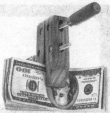

Drinking gourmet coffee may not be your particular vice, but if you take a good look at your budget, you'll probably find something that can be eliminated—or at the very least, cut back on. Maybe you'll have to cancel your $100/month satellite TV subscription. That would free up $1,200 a year that you could spend on prepping supplies. Maybe you can trade in your huge four-wheel drive Suburban for a gas-saving economy car. You could then use the money that you save on gas for prepping.

The point is that most people aren't really being honest with themselves when they say that there just isn't any room in the budget to start prepping. In most cases, with a little creative thinking, you can find some money to allocate to the prepping portion of your budget. It often really just depends on how badly you actually *want* to start prepping.

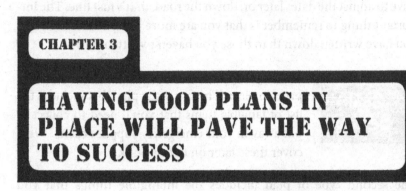

CHAPTER 3

HAVING GOOD PLANS IN PLACE WILL PAVE THE WAY TO SUCCESS

Soon we'll get into the meat and potatoes of this book and share some great prepping tips, but before we do that, let's talk about the importance of having good prepping plans in place.

It's very easy to get overwhelmed with everything that need to be done to successfully prepare for doomsday. Being overwhelmed will either lead to frantic unorganized prepping or doing nothing at all to prepare. Neither of these are good paths to take.

The best advice for now is to read through this book entirely. This will help you become familiar with the tasks that need to be done to prepare for doomsday. Then, take an afternoon to sit down and write a list of all the things you would like to do to prepare for doomsday. Write this list as if you had the money to go out and buy everything today. This will help make sure that you're not leaving items out because you're worried about how much everything will cost.

Once you have this list made out, it's time to break the list down into things that you can do right away. There will be plenty that you can do to prepare that won't cost much, if any, money at all. The simple fact that you are doing something to prepare will motivate you and inspire you to continue prepping. That's why it's so important to get started doing the little inexpensive things right away.

Next write down your mid-term goals and your long-term goals, being sure to include the dates that you would like to accomplish them. Don't be afraid to set goals because they are, in fact, only goals. If you have to adjust the dates later on down the road, that's just fine. The important thing to remember is that you are more likely to achieve goals you have written down than those you haven't written down.

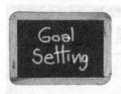

You're going to want to have a few different types of plans in place. The first is the plan that includes the list of tangible items that you'll need to collect to put away in your emergency supplies cache. We'll cover these later on in this book.

The second type of plan includes the intangible things that you should be doing to prepare for doomsday. These include increasing your knowledge, skills, and physical fitness so that when you eventually find yourself having to survive in a crisis, you'll be up for the challenge. We'll cover these topics later in this book, as well.

The third type of plan that you should have in place is your "bug out" plan. A bug out plan is ideal and necessary for times when it might become too dangerous to stay in your home. Depending upon where you live, you may plan to try to stay put and survive at home for as long as you can. In the prepping world, people call this "bugging in."

Regardless of how well you plan and prepare to bug in, you need to be prepared to get out of town if conditions become too dangerous at home. When it comes to bugging out, you should try to anticipate multiple scenarios, which means that you should have several evacu-

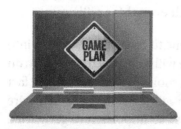

ation routes in mind. If you only have one planned evacuation route in mind and half a million other people happen to have the *same* idea, you'll find yourself wishing you had taken the time to include multiple evacuation routes in your planning.

Having these three types of plans in place will enable you to move forward as you prepare for doomsday and achieve your goals one by one. If you try to be a prepper without having well-thought-out plans in place, you'll find yourself wandering aimlessly as you gather a little here and there. Ultimately, you won't end up being nearly as prepared as you would have been if you had followed a set of detailed plans.

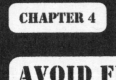

CHAPTER 4

AVOID FRUSTRATION BY STARTING WITH THE EASY THINGS FIRST

When getting started as a prepper, it's easy to focus too much on the "cool prepping gear." You might spend your time some days dreaming about that 2,000-square-foot underground survival bunker that you've always wanted to build.

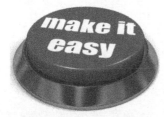

You may even fool yourself into believing that you're actually prepping by spending countless hours designing every last detail of your ideal emergency bunker. The reality is that you're not really doing anything to prepare unless you actually have the funds to follow through and install and build the bunker. If you don't have the money to follow through with this project, you're just daydreaming and wasting time. Instead of daydreaming about prepping, you should spend your time actually *doing* something that will help you survive when doomsday finally arrives.

A great example of an easy way to get started is storing water. As a matter of fact, one of the most important elements of any prepper's stockpile should be their water supply. Ironically, storing water is one of the least expensive and easiest things a prepper can do.

The main thing to keep in mind is that doing something is always better than doing nothing when it comes to prepping. Putting up water may not be as fun as dreaming up all the cool features that you would like to have in your ideal emergency bunker, but it needs to be done. And, best of all, it doesn't cost much money to do.

CHAPTER 5

HOW TO RECOGNIZE THE ARRIVAL OF DAY ONE

To some, Day One means the mushroom cloud on the horizon, the choking in the Tokyo subway, or trekking across subarctic areas in running shoes while the temperature plummets to −40°F. Wrong, that is *Day Two*! By that time, you should have been in a fallout shelter, avoiding the subway, or wearing insulated clothing and pulling a cargo toboggan.

To recognize Day One, you must be an armchair general, keeping abreast of the news and having the knowledge and equipment to muddle through Day Two. The only way to survive in style is to have a plan and the knowledge to carry it through. Day One can be anywhere from one day to ten years long, depending on the disaster scenario you are facing. In the individual scenarios, we will try to focus on their estimated duration.

Similarly, Day Two or Day Three are not necessarily of a twenty-four-hour duration. Perhaps it would have been more precise to call them phases. However, it is easier to think of them as days. When you look back upon an interesting phase of your life, you think of specific days while skipping over other intervening ones when nothing much happened. So it is with this book.

Day One is critical to your well-being. This is when you plan, prepare, accumulate supplies, and learn new skills to carry you through the following days. What you do on Day One determines whether you will live through any of the scenarios detailed in this book in style. Some people will survive without preparation by sheer luck, but that is not the way to bet. What you are betting is your existence and the existence of those you love.

Day One is unusual in that if you do not prepare for it, unless you are very lucky, you have lost the battle. Your planning starts when you realize that things can happen to you. Day One is the day when many people will ridicule you if they know that you are preparing for something. On the other hand, if you do not prepare, you are not likely to have any descendants. As the old saying goes, "If your parents did not have any children, you are not likely to have any either."

At the very least have your passport and other important papers up to date and close to you. What should you keep in your safety deposit box? Your fire insurance policy, copies of important papers, a copy of your last will, and similar documents. Do not keep cash, gold, firearms, or like items in your safety deposit box. Under many circumstances, they will get you into trouble. Even in a nonemergency situation, think what the IRS, the BATF, or the FBI would make of them.

Where should you keep the originals of your papers and your valuables? The answer depends on where you live. If your home is one room in a boardinghouse and your landlord regularly pokes around your place, the best solution is to carry your valuables with you, wherever you go. On the other hand, if you own a house in the suburbs, there are many more places to hide your valuables and supplies.

There is a tendency among us to brag a little about the preparations we make. I can't repeat it often enough—keeping a low profile is very important in this business. You may have an impromptu show-and-tell session with a neighbor, who doesn't believe there could be hard times. Once something does happen, he will turn on you for your supplies. His lack of preparedness is partially due to the government-encouraged belief that "it can't happen here." It will and you better be prepared for it, even if your neighbor isn't.

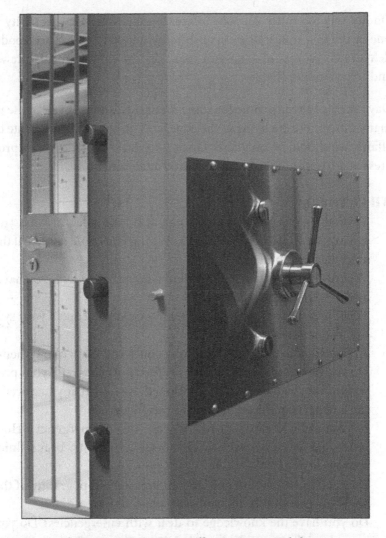

Except in a few cases, Day One will not arrive with large neon signs and sound effects proclaiming that it is here. In most cases, Day One arrives like a thief in the night. Sometimes it is only on Day Two that many will realize that Day One was yesterday. As a general piece of advice, assume that Day One is on hand now. Lay in supplies, learn new skills, and keep informed on what is happening in the world. Accumulate stocks of food that you eat now, and rotate those stocks.

Do not rely too much on your freezer and refrigerator. Electricity is one of the first things to go in an emergency. Rely on canned foods, dehydrated sachets of soup and pasta dishes, canned meats, stews, and other nonperishables.

Day One has already come for some scenarios, and it is very close to many others. We are living at the edge, and given the current state of affairs, we should be on guard. Once a scenario unfolds, it can progress at a frightening pace. Be prepared at all times.

WHAT TO DO:

- Take stock of what you are eating, and take stock of what you have on hand. That will tell you how long you could survive if the stores close tomorrow.
- Where do you get your water? Find what other sources you have, and have those sources tested.
- What happens to your sewage? How would you cope if your system is disrupted?
- Are you on medications? How long could you last without them? Do you have an alternate source for them? Always refill your prescriptions ahead of time. If questioned, just say that you are taking a trip. Have at least a month's supply on hand.
- Is your vehicle ready to roll in case of an emergency? How much gas do you have? What about lubricants, brake fluid, spare parts?
- Do you have a place to go? Do you know the topography of the area between your home and your place of retreat?
- Do you have the knowledge to deal with emergencies? Do you have the skills to put the knowledge into practice?
- How can you make your home harder to break into by criminals and looters?
- Can you handle firearms for self-defense? Do you have the firearms along with ammunition and spare parts to maintain them? Can you reload ammunition?
- Have you taken a first-aid course in the last five years? Do you have the supplies and instruments to give first aid?

- Are you aware of what is happening in your community, your country, and in the world? Do you have radios, communication devices, and newsletters to keep you informed?
- Do you have the financial or barter assets to start all over again?

A lot of hard questions are raised above. Yet, unless you sit down and answer them in the hard light of honesty, your chances of surviving even a temporary interruption in your present mode of life will be reduced.

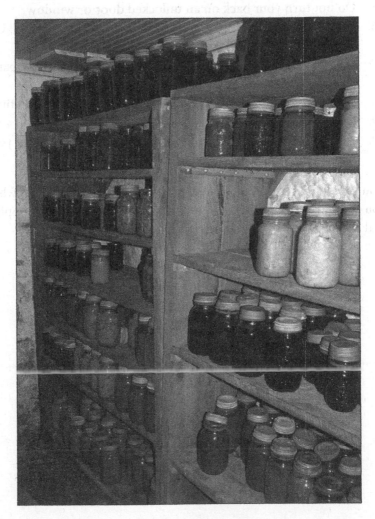

Then there is the question of security while you are preparing to survive. The ten commandments of security are:

1. Do not discuss personal or family business with anyone not directly involved.
2. Do not trust a politician or bureaucrat's word or promise.
3. Never give your real name or address when purchasing survival supplies.
4. Never let strangers into your home.
5. Do not turn your back on an unlocked door or window.
6. Do not have your street address on any of your IDs or mail. Use a P.O. box as much as you can.
7. Do not keep all your money or valuables in the same bank. Have several bank accounts under different names.
8. Never rely on someone else doing anything correctly or on time.
9. Do not have important mail sent to your home.
10. Always set the alarm and lock your garage when leaving your home.

You should be getting concerned by now. I would suggest that while you still have time, learn and practice new skills and lay in supplies and books. You must have the right psychology to survive.

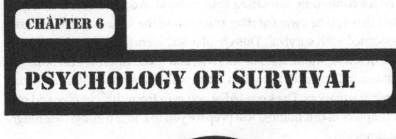

CHÀPTER 6

PSYCHOLOGY OF SURVIVAL

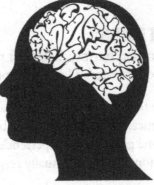

It takes much more than the knowledge and skills to build shelters, get food, make fires, and travel without the aid of standard navigational devices to live successfully through a survival situation. Some people with little or no survival training have managed to survive life-threatening circumstances. Some people with survival training have not used their skills and died. A key ingredient in any survival situation is the mental attitude of the individual(s) involved. Having survival skills is important; having the will to survive is essential. Without a desk to survive, acquired skills serve little purpose and invaluable knowledge goes to waste.

There is a psychology to survival. Finding yourself in a survival environment will produce many stresses that will have an impact on your mind. These stresses can produce thoughts and emotions that, if poorly understood, can even transform a confident, well-trained individual into an indecisive, ineffective individual with a questionable ability to survive. Therefore, you must be able to recognize those stresses commonly associated with survival. Additionally, it is imperative that you be aware of their reactions to the wide variety of stresses associated with survival. This chapter will identify and explain the nature of stress, the stresses of survival, and those internal reactions you will naturally experience when faced with the stresses of a real-world survival situation. The knowledge you gain from this chapter and other chapters in this manual will prepare you to come through the toughest times alive.

A LOOK AT STRESS

Before we can understand our psychological reactions in a survival setting, it is helpful to first know a little bit about stress.

Stress is not a disease that you cure and eliminate. Instead, it is a condition we all experience. Stress can be described as our reaction to pressure. It is the name given to the experience we have as we physically, mentally, emotionally, and spiritually respond to life's tensions.

NEED FOR STRESS

We need stress because it has many positive benefits. Stress provides us with challenges; it gives us chances to learn about our values and strengths. Stress can show our ability to handle pressure without breaking; it tests our adaptability and flexibility; it can stimulate us to do our best. Because we usually do not consider unimportant events stressful, stress can also be an excellent indicator of the significance we attach to an event—in other words, it highlights what is important to us.

We need to have some stress in our lives, but too much of anything can be bad. The goal is to have stress, but not an excess of it. Too much stress can take its toll on people and organizations. Too much stress leads to distress. Distress causes an uncomfortable tension that we try to escape and, preferably, avoid. Listed below are a few of the common signs of distress you may find in others or yourself when faced with too much stress:

- Difficulty making decisions.
- Angry outbursts.
- Forgetfulness.
- Low energy level.
- Constant worrying.
- Propensity for mistakes.
- Thoughts about death or suicide.
- Trouble getting along with others.
- Withdrawing from others.
- Hiding from responsibilities.
- Carelessness.

As you can see, stress can be constructive or destructive. It can encourage or discourage, move us along or stop us dead in our tracks, and make life meaningful or seemingly meaningless. Stress can inspire you to operate successfully and perform at your maximum efficiency in a survival situation. It can also cause you to panic and forget all your training. Key to your survival is your ability to manage the inevitable stresses you will encounter. The survivor is the person who works with his stresses instead of letting his stresses work on him.

SURVIVAL STRESSORS

Any event can lead to stress, and, as everyone has experienced, events don't always come one at a time. Often, stressful events occur simultaneously. These events are not stress, but they produce it and are called "stressors." Stressors are the obvious cause while stress is the response. Once the body recognizes the presence of a stressor, it then begins to act to protect itself.

In response to a stressor, the body prepares either to "fight or flee." This preparation involves an internal SOS sent throughout the body. As the body responds to this SOS, several actions take place. The body releases stored fuels (sugar and fats) to provide quick energy; breathing rate increases to supply more oxygen to the blood; muscle tension increases to prepare for action; blood clotting mechanisms are activated to reduce bleeding from cuts; senses become more acute (hearing becomes more sensitive, eyes become big, smell becomes sharper) so that you are more aware of your surroundings and heart rate and blood pressure rise to provide more blood to the muscles. This protective posture lets a person cope with potential dangers; however, a person cannot maintain such a level of alertness indefinitely.

Stressors are not courteous; one stressor does not leave because another one arrives. Stressors add up. The cumulative effect of minor stressors can be a major distress if they all happen too close together. As the body's resistance to stress wears down and the sources of stress continue (or increase), eventually a state of exhaustion arrives. At this point, the ability to resist stress or use it in a positive way gives out and signs of distress appear. Anticipating stressors and developing strategies to cope with them are two ingredients in the effective management of stress. It is therefore essential that, in a survival setting, you be aware of the types of stressors you will encounter. Let's take a look at a few of these.

INJURY, ILLNESS, OR DEATH
Injury, illness, and death are real possibilities a survivor has to face. Perhaps nothing is more stressful than being alone in an unfamiliar environment where you could die from an accident, or from eating something lethal. Illness and injury can also add to stress by limiting your ability to maneuver, get food and drink, find shelter, and defend yourself. Even if illness and injury don't lead to death, they add to stress through the pain and discomfort they generate. It is only by controlling the stress associated with the vulnerability to injury, illness, and death that you can have the courage to take the risks associated with survival tasks.

UNCERTAINLY AND LACK OF CONTROL
Some people have trouble operating in settings where everything

is not clear-cut. The only guarantee in a survival situation is that nothing is guaranteed. It can be extremely stressful operating on limited information in a setting where you have limited control of your surroundings. This uncertainty and lack of control also add to the stress of being ill, injured, or killed.

ENVIRONMENT
Even under the most ideal circumstances, nature is quite formidable. In survival, you will have to contend with the stressors of weather, terrain, and the variety of creatures inhabiting an area. Heat, cold, rain, winds, mountains, swamps, deserts, insects, dangerous reptiles, and other animals are just a few of the challenges awaiting you as you work to survive. Depending on how you handle the stress of your environment, your surroundings can be either a source of food and protection or can be a cause of extreme discomfort leading to injury, illness, or death.

HUNGER AND THIRST
Without food and water a person will weaken and eventually die. Thus, getting and preserving food and water takes on increasing importance as the length of time in a survival setting increases. For someone used to getting food in a supermarket, foraging can be a big source of stress.

FATIGUE
Forcing yourself to continue surviving is not easy as you grow more tired. It is possible to become so fatigued that the act of just staying awake is stressful in itself.

ISOLATION
There are some advantages to facing adversity with others. While we may learn survival skills as individuals, all people are naturally

communal, especially during times of confusion. Being in contact with others also provides a greater sense of security and a feeling that someone is available to help if problems occur. A significant stressor in survival situations is that often a person or team has to rely solely on its own resources.

The survival stressors mentioned in this section are by no means the only ones you may face. Remember, what is stressful to one person may not be stressful to another. Your experiences, training, personal outlook on life, physical and mental conditioning, and level of self-confidence contribute to what you will find stressful in a survival environment. The object is not to avoid stress, but rather to manage the stressors of survival and make them work for you.

We now have a general knowledge of stress and the stressors common to survival; the next step is to examine our reactions to the stressors we may face.

NATURAL REACTIONS

Man has been able to survive many shifts in his environment throughout the centuries. His ability to adapt physically and mentally to a changing world kept him alive while other species around him gradually died off. The same survival mechanisms that kept our forefathers alive can help keep us alive as well! However, these survival mechanisms that can help us can also work against us if we don't understand and anticipate their presence.

It is not surprising that the average person will have some psychological reactions in a survival situation. We will now examine some of the major internal reactions you and anyone with you might experience with the survival stressors addressed in the earlier paragraphs. Let's begin.

FEAR

Fear is our emotional response to dangerous circumstances that we believe have the potential to cause death, injury, or illness. This harm is not just limited to physical damage; the threat to one's emotional and mental well-being can generate fear as well. For a person trying to survive, fear can have a positive function if it encourages him to be cautious in situations where recklessness could result in injury. Unfortunately, fear can also immobilize a person. It can cause him to become so frightened that he fails to perform activities essential for survival. Most people will have some degree of fear when placed in unfamiliar surroundings under adverse conditions. There is no shame in this! Everyone must train himself not to be overcome by his fears. Ideally, through realistic training, we can acquire the knowledge and skills needed to increase our confidence and thereby manage our fears.

ANXIETY

Associated with fear is anxiety. Because it is natural for us to be afraid, it is also natural for us to experience anxiety. Anxiety can be an uneasy, apprehensive feeling we get when faced with dangerous situations (physical, mental, and emotional). When used in a healthy way, anxiety urges us to act to end, or at least master, the dangers that threaten our existence. If we were never anxious, there would be little motivation to make changes in our lives. In a survival setting, we can reduce our anxiety by performing those tasks that will ensure we come through the ordeal alive. As we reduce our anxiety, we also bring under control the source of that anxiety—our fears. In this form, anxiety is good; however, anxiety can also have a devastating impact. Anxiety can overwhelm a person to the point where he becomes easily confused and has difficulty thinking. Once this happens, it becomes more and more difficult for him to make good judgments and sound decisions. To survive, we must learn techniques to calm our anxieties and keep them in the range where they help, not hurt.

ANGER AND FRUSTRATION

Frustration arises when a person is continually thwarted in his attempts to reach a goal. The goal of survival is to stay alive until you can reach help or until help can reach you. To achieve this goal, you

must complete some tasks with minimal resources. It is inevitable, in trying to do these tasks, that something will go wrong; that something will happen beyond your control; and that with one's life at stake, every mistake is magnified in terms of its importance. Thus, sooner or later, we will have to cope with frustration when a few of our plans run into trouble. One outgrowth of this frustration is anger. There are many events in a survival situation that can frustrate or anger you. Getting lost, damaged or forgotten equipment, the weather, inhospitable terrain, and physical limitations are just a few sources of frustration and anger. Frustration and anger encourage impulsive reactions, irrational behavior, poorly thought-out decisions, and, in some instances, an "I quit" attitude (people sometimes avoid doing something they can't master). If you can harness and properly channel the emotional intensity associated with anger and frustration, you can productively act as you answer the challenges of survival. If you do not properly focus your angry feelings, you can waste much energy in activities that do little to further either your chances of survival or the chances of those around you.

DEPRESSION

It would be a rare person indeed who would not get sad, at least momentarily, when faced with the privations of survival. As this sadness deepens, we label the feeling "depression." Depression is closely linked with frustration and anger. The frustrated person becomes more and more angry as he fails to reach his goals. If the anger does not help the person to succeed, then the frustration level goes even higher. A destructive cycle between anger and frustration continues until the person becomes worn down—physically, emotionally, and mentally. When a person reaches this point, he starts to give up, and his focus shifts from "What can I do?" to "There is nothing I can do." Depression is an expression of this hopeless, helpless feeling. There is nothing wrong with being sad as you temporarily think about your loved ones and remember what life is like back in "civilization" or "the world." Such thoughts, in fact, can give you the desire to try harder and live one more day. On the other hand, if you allow yourself to sink into a depressed state, then it can sap all your energy and, more important, your will to survive. It is imperative that you resist succumbing to depression.

LONELINESS AND BOREDOM

Man is a social animal. This means we, as human beings, enjoy the company of others. Very few people want to be alone *all the time!* As you are aware, there is a distinct chance of isolation in a survival setting. This is not bad. Loneliness and boredom can bring to the surface qualities you thought only others had. The extent of your imagination and creativity may surprise you. When required to do so, you may discover some hidden talents and abilities. Most of all, you may tap into a reservoir of inner strength and fortitude you never knew you had. Conversely, loneliness and boredom can be another source of depression. As a person surviving alone, or with others, you must find ways to keep your mind productively occupied. Additionally, you must develop a degree of self-sufficiency. You must have faith in your capability to "go it alone."

GUILT

The circumstances leading to your being in a survival setting are sometimes dramatic and tragic. It may be the result of an accident where there was a loss of life. Perhaps you were the only, or one of a few, survivors. While naturally relieved to be alive, you simultaneously may be mourning the deaths of others who were less fortunate. It is not uncommon for survivors to feel guilty about being spared from death while others were not. This feeling, when used in a positive way, has encouraged people to try harder to survive with the belief they were allowed to live for some greater purpose in life. Sometimes, survivors tried to stay alive so that they could carry on the work of those killed. Whatever reason you give yourself, do not let guilt feelings prevent you from living. The living who abandon their chance to survive accomplish nothing. Such an act would be the greatest tragedy.

PREPARING YOURSELF

Your task in a survival situation is to stay alive. As you can see, you are going to experience an assortment of thoughts and emotions. These can work for you, or they can work to your downfall. Fear, anxiety, anger, frustration, guilt, depression, and loneliness are all possible reactions to the many stresses common to survival. These reactions, when controlled in a healthy way, help to increase your likelihood of surviving. They prompt you to pay more attention in training, to fight back when scared, to take actions that ensure sustenance and security, to keep faith with your fellows, and to strive against large odds. When the survivor cannot control these reactions in a healthy way, they can bring him to a standstill. Instead of rallying his internal resources, he listens to his internal fears. This person will experience psychological defeat long before he physically succumbs. Remember, survival is natural to everyone; being unexpectedly thrust into the life and death struggle of survival is not. Don't be afraid of your "natural reactions to this unnatural situation." Prepare yourself to rule over these reactions so they serve your ultimate interest—staying alive.

It involves preparation to ensure that your reactions in a survival setting are productive, not destructive. The challenge of survival has produced countless examples of heroism, courage, and self-sacrifice. These are the qualities it can bring out in you if you have prepared yourself. Below are a few tips to help prepare yourself psychologically for survival. Through studying this manual and attending survival training you can develop the *survival attitude.*

KNOW YOURSELF
Through training, family, and friends take the time to discover who you are on the inside. Strengthen your stronger qualities and develop the areas that you know are necessary to survive.

ANTICIPATE FEARS
Don't pretend that you will have no fears. Begin thinking about what would frighten you the most if forced to survive alone. Train in those areas of concern to you. The goal is not to eliminate the fear, but to build confidence in your ability to function despite your fears.

BE REALISTIC

Don't be afraid to make an honest appraisal of situations. See circumstances as they are, not as you want them to be. Keep your hopes and expectations within the estimate of the situation. When you go into a survival setting with unrealistic expectations, you may be laying the groundwork for bitter disappointment.

Follow the adage, "Hope for the best, prepare for the worst." It is much easier to adjust to pleasant surprises about one's unexpected good fortunes than to be upset by one's unexpected harsh circumstances.

ADOPT A POSITIVE ATTITUDE

Learn to see the potential good in everything. Looking for the good not only boosts morale, it also is excellent for exercising your imagination and creativity.

REMIND YOURSELF WHAT IS AT STAKE

Remember, failure to prepare yourself psychologically to cope with survival leads to reactions such as depression, carelessness, inattention, loss of confidence, poor decision-making, and giving up before the body gives in. At stake is your life and the lives of others who are depending on you to do your share.

TRAIN

Through training and life experiences, begin today to prepare yourself to cope with the rigors of survival. Demonstrating your skills in training will give you the confidence to call upon them should the need arise. Remember, the more realistic the training, the less overwhelming an actual survival setting will be.

LEARN STRESS MANAGEMENT TECHNIQUES

People under stress have a potential to panic if they are not well trained and not prepared psychologically to face whatever the circumstances may be. While we often cannot control the survival circumstances in which we find ourselves, it is within our ability to control our response to those circumstances. Learning stress management techniques can enhance significantly your capability to remain calm and focused as you work to keep yourself and others alive. A few good techniques to develop include relaxation skills, time management skills, assertiveness skills, and cognitive restructuring skills (the ability to control how you view a situation).

Remember, "the will to survive" can also be considered to be "the refusal to give up."

CHAPTER 7

EMERGENCY PREPAREDNESS

We usually don't want to wish trouble upon ourselves, but the possibility of facing a major or minor natural or man-made disaster is always present. It is always a good idea to learn how to protect yourself and cope with disaster by planning ahead; when disaster strikes you may not have much time to act.
Take time to learn about the potential hazards that may occur in your region and find out about your community's disaster response plans and procedures for warning and evacuation. Above all, take basic, sensible precautions and learn what to do if you face an emergency.

EMERGENCY PLANS

Create a plan for the family.

- Find the safe locations in your home for each type of disaster you may have to face.
- Make sure all family members, including children, know how and when to call 911, police and fire, and post emergency telephone numbers near telephones.
- Discuss what to do about power outages and teach family members how to turn off the water, gas, and electricity at main switches when necessary.
- Pick two emergency meeting places: A place near your home and a place outside your neighborhood in case you cannot return home after a disaster.

- Find out about your children's school emergency plan and monitor local media broadcasts for directions from local emergency officials' announcements about changes in school openings and closings. In cases where schools initiate shelter-in-place procedures, you may not be permitted to pick up your children; the school doors will probably be locked for safety.

FAMILY COMMUNICATION PLAN

In case family members are separated from one another during a disaster, create a plan for getting back together. Find an out-of-state relative or friend to serve as an emergency contact (it is frequently easier to call out-of-state than within the affected area) and be sure that everyone knows the name, address, and phone number of the contact. Make sure that every family member knows family and emergency contact numbers:

- 911, police, fire, hospital
- Alternate phone numbers or family members (work, cell, pager, etc.)
- Neighbors' names and telephone numbers
- Electric, gas, and water companies

EVACUATION PLAN

Plan ahead where to go and what to take with you if you are forced to leave. Making plans at the last minute is sure to cause panic and confusion. If community evacuation becomes necessary, local officials will provide evacuation warnings and instructions via local radio and television broadcasts. In some locations, other warning methods such as sirens or telephone calls are used.

Remember, it is vital to plan ahead. The amount of time you have to evacuate will depend on the type of emergency you face. In some potential disaster situations, a hurricane that can be monitored for example, you might have several days to prepare, but in other situations, such as a chemical release or flash flood, there may be no time to assemble even the most basic necessities.

HOUSEHOLD ESCAPE PLAN

In some emergencies, you may need to get out of your home fast. Work out an escape plan by drawing a floor plan of your dwelling that shows the location of doors, windows, stairways and items of large furniture. Show the location of emergency supplies—fire extinguishers, collapsible ladders, first-aid kits and utility shut-off points. Chart at least two escape routes from each room. Designate a place outside of the home where everyone should meet.

SAFETY SKILLS

- Learn first aid and take a CPR class. Your local American Red Cross chapter can provide this type of training and certification.
- Be sure that everyone knows how to use a fire extinguisher and where it is kept.
- Review potential disaster scenarios in your area and learn how to take personal protection measures—where to seek shelter, when to duck and cover.

DISASTER SUPPLY KITS

Review what disasters you might face and assemble any emergency supplies you might need to store in your household or for an evacuation. Store them in easy-to-find places and keep evacuation supplies in a portable container such as a backpack or duffle bag. Make sure you have the tools you need to deal with any emergency.

FIRE EXTINGUISHERS

Fire extinguishers are your first line of defense against fire. Selecting the proper extinguisher is important to ensure that you have the right kind for the expected type of fire and to reduce damage to valuables caused by extinguishing agents. Make sure everyone knows the location, use, and limitations of your fire extinguishers. Extinguishers should be checked and serviced once a year.

Selecting a Fire Extinguisher

Extinguishers are classified according to the type of fire for which they are suitable.

- **Class A:** Ordinary combustibles—wood, paper, cloth, and most plastics.
- **Class B:** Flammable liquids and gases—gasoline, oils, paint, lacquers, and greases.
- **Class C:** Live electrical equipment—extinguishingagent must be nonconductive.

Extinguishers also have a numerical rating indicating the amount of fire the extinguisher will handle. The minimum rating for a Class A extinguisher to be used on minor hazards is 2A. For Class B or C hazards, a rating of 10 is the minimum size recommended. Some have combined ratings.

Extinguishing Agents:

- **Dry Chemical—Standard:** Useful on Class B and C fires (automotive, grease fires, and flammable liquids). Leaves a mildly corrosive residue that can damage electrical equipment.
- **Dry Chemical—Multipurpose:** Useful for Class A, B, and C fires. Effective on most common fires. Highly corrosive with sticky residue. Not for use around electrical appliances or computers.
- **Halogenated Agents:** Useful on Class A, B, and C fires (check labels for specifics). Mildly toxic but versatile, and leaves no residue.
- **Carbon Dioxide:** Useful on Class B and C fires. Very clean with no residue but are heavy, short range and must be applied close to fire.
- **Water-Based Agent:** Use on Class A fires only. These are inexpensive to refill and maintain.

REMEMBER: If an extinguisher is used, you should still call the fire department and evacuate the area. Fire personnel will make sure that the fire is out.

FAMILY RECORDS

Store your important documents and family records—deeds, property records, insurance policies, and other important papers—in a safe place such as a safety-deposit box or in a waterproof and fireproof container at home. Make copies of your important documents for your disaster supply kit. Important documents include:

- Driver's license and personal identification
- Passports
- Birth certificates
- Social Security cards
- Deeds and ownership certificates (automobiles, boats, etc.)
- Insurance policies along with your agent's contact information
- Wills
- Current photographs of family members
- Year, model, license plate number, and identification numbers (VIN) of vehicles
- Bank and financial account numbers with the appropriate contact information
- Lease and name and contact information for your landlord or property manager
- Important medical information (allergies, medications, and medical history)

PERSONAL PROPERTY INVENTORY

Make a record of your personal property for insurance purposes. Take photos or a video of the interior and exterior of your home. Include important personal belongings in your photo inventory.

INSURANCE

If you live in an area that is prone to certain natural hazards—hurricanes, earthquakes, etc.—review your insurance policies and determine what provisions and exemptions may apply to your situation. Household insurance policies generally exclude flood damage from rising water and other specific losses that can occur in the aftermath of a natural disaster. A policy may provide funds to rebuild your home, for example, but not cover the removal of damaged trees from your own property.

If you live in a flood-prone area, consider purchasing flood insurance. Flood insurance that covers the value of a building and its contents will not only provide greater peace of mind but will speed recovery. Be prepared by finding out how you are covered and what you might need to do to secure additional protection.

DIGITAL SURVIVAL—HOME BUSINESS AND COMPUTERS

Home businesses and individuals have come to rely on computers for everything from basic recordkeeping to financial management and tax preparation. Computers, however, are vulnerable to the effects of natural disasters such as power surges or failure and water damage. Data stored on computers can be corrupted or, worse, lost.

By preparing ahead for a potential disaster, you should be able to resume a home business without serious disruption. Take stock of the risks your business might face and make a plan to deal with those risks. Review your plan annually or when changes occur in the business to keep it current.

PROTECT YOUR HARDWARE

- Use a surge protector or an uninterrupted power supply backup to protect data in the event of a power outage. Replace surge protectors at least once a year.
- Keep your computer hardware and software licenses up to date. Maintain hardcopy records such as leases in a secure location.
- Have waterproof tarps to cover computers and equipment in case of water infiltration, and elevate and secure your equipment.

BACK UP YOUR FILES

Protect your vital business and personal records. Back up your data and create a plan to regularly back up your data and protect the backup. Include your key business information—budgets, client lists, sales and tax records, insurance, loans, and banking information. Keep important papers in a safety-deposit box and copies at another safe location.

- Make backups of any business or personal computer files—tax, accounting, production records, inventory, and customer lists.
- Back up your computer data automatically on a daily basis. Check the backup log regularly to ensure that backups are completed properly. Note that there are online remote backup services available.
- Use a removable or portable data storage device and back up your on-site data to it daily. If you must evacuate, you can easily take it with you.
- Protect your backups by keeping a set of backup files stored off-site and maintain permanent monthly archives. Store these file copies on an off-site server at least 50 miles away from your home or office.

INVENTORIES
- Keep an inventory of all hardware and software with serial, license and model numbers, and company information for leased or purchased hardware and software.
- Keep contact information for the company where you store off-site backups—include contact names and numbers.
- Record the serial and license numbers of all secondary computer devices (printers, hard drives, scanners, etc.).

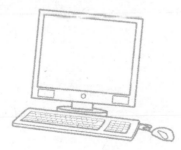

CHAPTER 8

EVACUATION

There are some situations where it is just too dangerous to try and ride out a natural disaster at home. State authorities often call upon residents of the Gulf Coast and Atlantic seaboard to evacuate their homes and businesses in the face of powerful hurricanes. In addition, transportation  and industrial accidents can result in the release of harmful chemicals, forcing the evacuation of entire neighborhoods. Wildfires, particularly in the western states, and flooding frequently cause hasty evacuations.

When such disasters strike, emergency management officials will provide evacuation information to the public via local radio and television broadcasts and by using the National Emergency Broadcasting System. If local officials ask you to evacuate, do so immediately. Depending on the situation, the amount of time you have to evacuate will vary. A hurricane may allow several days to prepare for an evacuation, while other situations, such as a hazardous material spill or chemical release, may allow only moments to get away.

Advanced planning will make any evacuation easier. Contact your local emergency management office to learn about the possible dangers in your area ahead of time, and find out about emergency warning systems along with evacuation routes and plans. Consider assembling a family disaster supply kit and make an evacuation plan. Remember, an evacuation can last for several days or longer and during that time you may be responsible for part or all of your own food, clothing, and other supplies.

PREPARE FOR EVACUATION

- Find out about evacuation plans for your community.
- Prepare a disaster supply kit. *(See Disaster Supply Kits, page 48.)*
- Discuss possible evacuation procedures with your family and make sure that everyone knows what to do.
- Plan a destination outside the potential disaster area in advance and get a map of the area.
- Locate the public emergency shelters in your region.
- Establish a check-in contact—a friend or relative outside your area—so that everyone in the family can call in to report that he is safe. Make sure all family members have that phone number.
- Find out where children will be sent if they are evacuated from their school.
- Keep a full tank of gas in your car if an evacuation seems likely. Gasoline may be unobtainable during a major evacuation.
- If you do not own a car or other vehicle, make arrangements for transportation with a friend, or contact your local emergency management office. Public transportation systems may not be available during an emergency.
- Make plans for pets and other domestic animals.
- Know how to shut off electricity, gas, and water at the main switches and valves. Make sure you have the tools you need (usually pipe and crescent or adjustable wrenches). Contact your local utility providers for additional information.

EVACUATION SUPPLIES

Assemble any supplies that you might need if you were to be away from home for several days and place them in an easy-to-carry container.

Label the container clearly and keep it in a designated, easily accessible place. Remember to include all of the disaster supply kit basics. You might consider assembling a car kit to keep in your vehicle that contains emergency supplies in case you are stranded; include flares, jumper cables, and seasonal supplies in addition to your disaster supply kit.

If ordered to evacuate:
- Listen to a battery-powered radio for evacuation instructions.
- Take your disaster supply kit with you if you are ordered to evacuate.
- Wear sturdy shoes and clothing that will provide some protection, such as long pants, long-sleeved shirts, and a cap or hat.
- Follow the recommended evacuation routes.
- Stay away from downed power lines.
- In a flooding situation, watch out for washed-out roads and bridges. Never try to drive through flooded roadways or bridges—find another way around.

If you have time:
- Let others know where you plan to go and leave a note telling when you left and your destination.
- Close and lock doors and windows.
- Unplug electrical appliances—radios, televisions, freezers, refrigerators, toasters, and microwaves.
- Make arrangements for pets.
- Shut off water, gas, and electricity and secure propane tanks before leaving, if instructed to do so.

If you have to leave immediately, take:
- Medical supplies: prescriptions and other necessary medications.
- Disaster supplies: flashlight, batteries, radio, first-aid kit, bottled water.
- Clothing and bedding: a change of clothing and a sleeping bag or bedroll for each member of the household.

PAPERS AND DOCUMENTS

You may want to consider consolidating important records and storing them in a safe, portable container. Make sure that your container is waterproof—a file box, plastic tub or box, or even sealable plastic freezer bags. If lost, these records may be difficult and time-consuming to replace.

- Driver's license, passport, or other personal identification
- Social Security cards
- A supply of cash
- Checkbook and credit cards (credit card and bank account information)
- Birth and marriage certificates
- Immunization records
- Proof of residence (deed or lease)
- Insurance policies (home, renters, auto, life, etc.)
- Wills and contracts
- Copies of recent tax returns

RETURNING HOME AFTER THE DISASTER

- Monitor radio and television broadcasts for information and instructions.
- Telephone your family and friends as soon as possible to tell them you are safe.
- Do not return until the local authorities confirm that it is safe.
- Do not reenter the house until authorities tell you it is safe to do so.
- Use caution when entering buildings that may have been damaged or weakened.
- Use a battery-operated flashlight or glow stick for light. Do not use exposed flame light sources in damaged buildings. There is a danger of flammable materials and leaking gas.
- If you suspect a gas leak or if you smell gas, leave the house immediately and notify the gas company or the fire department. Do not turn on the lights; a spark from the switch might ignite the gas.
- Notify the power company or fire department if you see damaged electrical wires.

- If any of your appliances are wet, turn off the main electrical power switch before attempting to unplug them. Dry all appliances, wall switches, and sockets thoroughly before you reconnect them.
- Check all food supplies for spoilage or contamination.
- Do not drink local water until it has been certified safe.
- Wear sturdy shoes or boots and use heavy gloves when handling debris.
- Watch for venomous snakes in flooded structures and debris.

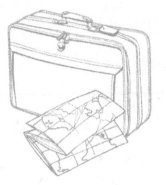

CHAPTER 9

PROJECT: BUG OUT BAG (BOB)

Personally, it would take a very severe reason for me to evacuate or "bug out" from my home in the first place. Leaving the house would entail me having to leave many of my in-place systems and make me more vulnerable to outlaws and well-meaning (and not so well-meaning) bureaucrats.

However, just because I don't *want* to evacuate from my homestead doesn't mean I won't *have* to evacuate. I don't want any kind of disaster to befall my family, but measuring risk says I should be prepared "just in case." This leads me to the subject of disaster evacuation kits.

Any prepper or interested party with access to the Internet has probably noticed the love of acronyms as they relate to kits and gear. You have BOB, INCH, GOOD, GHB, EDC, IFAK, 72-hour kits, and 1st, 2nd, and 3rd line gear. The confusion just piles on.

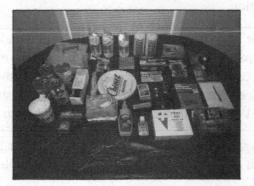

The reality is, it's pretty simple: It's all related to the things you need to survive under different scenarios. The concept of a 72-hour kit comes from the US military and is based on the fact that American soldiers are resupplied so often that they only need to be self-sufficient for three days at a time. This level is what the US government recommends for all citizens, because in the event of a federally declared disaster it will take FEMA approximately three days to get a supply system organized to provide relief. A 72-hour kit should have basic cooking, lighting, shelter, water, and food to survive for three days.

EDC, or "Everyday Carry," means the things you have on your body every day. BOB, bob, or B.o.B means "Bug Out Bag." A BOB is a small bag that is basically a portable 72-hour kit. The idea is that if a fire or something broke out and you had to leave *right now*, you can throw on your shoes, grab your BOB, and have whatever essential medicines, food, and clothes you would need. A good idea is to have copies of vital records in your BOB (project 1), so that you won't lose them if you don't have time to dig around in your filing cabinet.

A GHB, or "Get Home Bag," is practically the same as a BOB, but philosophically the opposite. A GHB is a portable kit containing the essentials you would need if you had to find an alternate route home if disaster struck while you were away from home. I keep a GHB in my vehicle, as well as my wife's. Due to the nature of cars, my GHB is actually a box that has a lot of stuff for light repairs, minimalist camping, and a walk home. Space and weight are not issues in the car, so I have things in my box that I can pick through to make a bag that best fits my situation.

Many people keep firearms in their GHBs and I understand that; however, if you have an assault rifle or other long arm and change into a multi-cam "uniform," you're going to attract unwanted attention. Consider a more concealable approach to defensive weaponry. In a disaster I want to blend in until I have to stand out.

A GOOD bag, or "Get Out Of Dodge" bag, is a larger BOB, but still small enough to carry. It's pretty much interchangeable with a BOB, just larger in scope. Some preppers have GOOD trailers or GOOD vehicles that are pre-packed. I use big plastic totes with a color code system.

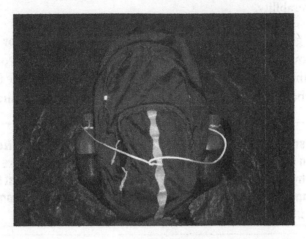

An INCH bag stands for "I'm Never Coming Home." It's more of a Mad Max/*The Road*/*The Postman* type problem where you have to take what you can carry, but all you own is what you take. My INCH bag would contain everything in my GOOD kit, plus extras like my hand-reloading press, more tools, and some small reference materials.

IFAK is an "Individual First Aid Kit," also known as an "Improved First Aid Kit" depending on the branch of service. This individual kit is part of a new military soldier initiative. It's a one-pound kit that addresses major blood loss and airway distress.

Line gear is also a military concept and centers around the gear you would need to complete a mission. It's not exactly applicable to citizen preppers, but it is related.

1st line gear is your EDC and focuses on what you would carry on your person. This would include your clothing, knife, weapon and, maybe a small survival and first aid kit.

2nd line gear is your "fighting load," which for me fits in a messenger bag. In this bag I can carry items like a flashlight, a hand-held radio, batteries, and calorie-dense energy bars. It also can go with me almost everywhere and gives me more capability without sacrificing a lot of maneuverability.

3rd line gear is your pack—sustainment items you need for a longer term. You're not going to fight wearing your rucksack; you would drop it and depend on your 1st and 2nd line gear during the fight and then go back and get your pack to refill your empty magazines.

It doesn't matter if you use the "proper" terms; just organize your gear to suit your needs. As long as you understand what you're doing and why you're doing it, you are light years ahead of guys that follow the conventional prepper wisdom and build kits based upon what some Internet guru wrote in a list.

It is important that you take some time to develop a plan that fits into your personal situation. All things being equal, less gear that you can use well and have on you is better than lots of gear you cannot use and do not carry.

That being said, today's project is to look around the house and assemble a small 72-hour kit to get you by until you finish your incremental disaster kit. Put in this kit everything you would need to survive 72 hours using the contents of this kit alone. Then schedule a weekend to try it out. Turn off the power and the water and see exactly how hard it is. This will show you the weaknesses of your kit, while putting you in a situation that could happen after a large winter storm or other natural disaster.

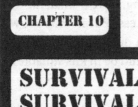

CHAPTER 10

SURVIVAL PLANNING AND SURVIVAL KITS

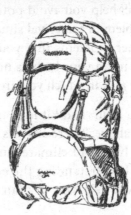

Survival planning is nothing more than realizing something could happen that would put you in a survival situation and, with that in mind, taking steps to increase your chances of survival. Thus, survival planning means preparation.

Preparation means having survival items and knowing how to use them. People who live in snow regions prepare their vehicles for poor road conditions. They put snow tires on their vehicles, add extra weight in the back for traction, and they carry a shovel, salt, and a blanket. Another example of preparation is finding the emergency exits on an aircraft when you board it for a flight. Preparation could also mean knowing your intended route of travel and familiarizing yourself with the area. Finally, emergency planning is essential.

IMPORTANCE OF PLANNING

Detailed prior planning is essential in potential survival situations. Including survival considerations will enhance your chances of survival if an emergency occurs. Your ability to carry survival items on your person is usually limited. When traveling, have a small kit with selected items that is always within easy access. Put it where it will not prevent you from getting out of the area quickly, yet where it is readily accessible. Bulky and heavy items should be in kits suitable for vehicles or boats.

One important aspect of prior planning is preventive medicine. Ensuring that you have no dental problems and that your immunizations are current will help you avoid potential dental or health problems. A dental problem in a survival situation will reduce your ability to cope with other problems that you face. Failure to keep your shots current may mean your body is not immune to diseases that are prevalent in the area in which you are traveling.

Preparing and carrying a survival kit is as important as the considerations mentioned above. There are kits for overwater survival, for hot climate survival, cold climate survival, survival in the mountains and desert. Understanding the environment in which you will be traveling will help you to plan and to prepare your own survival kit.

Even the smallest survival kit, if properly prepared, is invaluable when faced with a survival problem. Before making your survival kit, however, consider the environment, the terrain, the weather, and your ability to carry or transport your kit.

SURVIVAL KITS

The environment is the key to the types of items you will need in your survival kit. How much equipment you put in your kit depends on how you will carry the kit. A kit carried on your body will have to be smaller than one carried in a vehicle. Always layer your survival kit, keeping the most important items on your body. For example, your map and compass should always be on your body. Carry less important items in your pack. Place bulky items in your vehicle.

In preparing your survival kit, remember that size and weight is critical, and select items you can use for more than one purpose. If you have two items that will serve the same function, pick the one you can use for another function. Do not duplicate items, as this increases your kit's size and weight.

Your survival kit need not be elaborate. You need only functional items that will meet your needs and a case to hold the items. For the case, you might want to use a Band-Aid box, a first aid case, an ammunition pouch, or another suitable case. This case should be:

- Water repellent or waterproof.
- Easy to carry or attach to your body.
- Suitable to accept varisized components.
- Durable.

In your survival kit, you should have:

- First aid items.
- Water purification tablets/drops or preferably a compact portable filtration system.
- Fire starting equipment.
- Signaling items.
- Food procurement items.
- Shelter items.

Some examples of these items are:

- Lighter, metal match, waterproof matches.
- Snare wire.
- Signaling mirror.
- Wrist compass.
- Fish and snare line.
- Fishhooks.

- Candle.
- Small hand lens.
- Oxytetracycline tablets (diarrhea or infection).
- Water purification tablets or a compact, reusable filtration device.
- Solar blanket.
- Surgical blades.
- Butterfly sutures.
- Condoms for water storage.
- Chap Stick.
- Needle and thread.
- Knife.
- Hatchet.

Include a firearm only if the situation so dictates. Firearms require ammunition and both can be heavy. Read about and practice the survival techniques in this manual. Then prepare your survival kit.

SHELTER SITE SELECTION

CHAPTER 11

SHELTERS

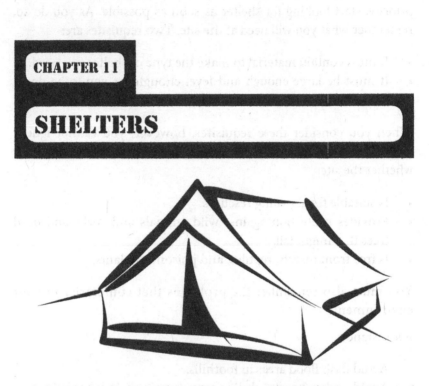

A shelter can protect you from the sun, insects, wind, rain, snow, and hot or cold temperatures. It can give you a feeling of well-being. It can help you maintain your will to survive.

In some areas, your need for shelter may take precedence over your need for food and possibly even your need for water. For example, prolonged exposure to cold can cause excessive fatigue and weakness (exhaustion). An exhausted person may develop a "passive" outlook, thereby losing the will to survive.

The most common error in making a shelter is to make it too large. A shelter must be large enough to protect you. It must also be small enough to contain your body heat, especially in cold climates.

SHELTER SITE SELECTION

When you are in a survival situation and realize that shelter is a high priority, start looking for shelter as soon as possible. As you do so, remember what you will need at the site. Two requisites are:

- It must contain material to make the type of shelter you need.
- It must be large enough and level enough for you to lie down comfortably.

When you consider these requisites, however, you cannot ignore other factors contributing to your safety. You must also consider whether the site:

- Is suitable for signaling rescuers.
- Provides protection against wild animals and rocks and dead trees that might fall.
- Is free from insects, reptiles, and poisonous plants.

You must also remember the problems that could arise in your environment.

For instance:

- Avoid flash flood areas in foothills.
- Avoid avalanche or rockslide areas in mountainous terrain.
- Avoid sites near bodies of water that are below the high water mark.

In some areas, the season of the year has a strong bearing on the site you select. Ideal sites for a shelter differ in winter and summer. During cold winter months you will want a site that will protect you from the cold and wind, but will have a source of fuel and water. During summer months in the same area you will want a source of water, but you will want the site to be almost insect free.

TYPES OF SHELTERS

When looking for a shelter site, keep in mind the type of shelter (protection) you need. However, you must also consider:

- How much time and effort you need to build the shelter.
- If the shelter will adequately protect you from the elements (sun, wind, rain, snow).
- If you have the tools to build it. If not, can you make improvised tools?
- If you have the type and amount of materials needed to build it.

To answer these questions, you need to know how to make various types of shelters and what materials you need to make them.

PONCHO LEAN-TO

It takes only a short time and minimal equipment to build this lean-to. You need a poncho, 2 to 3 meters of rope or parachute suspension line, three stakes about 30 centimeters long, and two trees or two poles 2 to 3 meters apart. Before selecting the trees you will use or the location of your poles, check the wind direction. Ensure that the back of your lean-to will be into the wind.

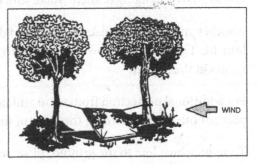

Poncho lean-to.

To make the lean-to:

- Tie off the hood of the poncho. Pull the drawstring tight, roll the hood longways, fold it into thirds, and tie it off with the drawstring.
- Cut the rope in half. On one long side of the poncho, tie half of the rope to the corner grommet. Tie the other half to the other corner grommet.
- Attach a drip stick (about a 10-centimeter stick) to each rope about 2.5 centimeters from the grommet. These drip sticks will keep rainwater from running down the ropes into the lean-to. Tying strings (about 10 centimeters long) to each grommet along

53

the poncho's top edge will allow the water to run to and down the line without dripping into the shelter.

- Tie the ropes about waist high on the trees (uprights). Use a round turn and two half hitches with a quick-release knot.
- Spread the poncho and anchor it to the ground, putting sharpened sticks through the grommets and into the ground.

If you plan to use the lean-to for more than one night, or you expect rain, make a center support for the lean-to. Make this support with a line. Attach one end of the line to the poncho hood and the other end to an overhanging branch. Make sure there is no slack in the line.

Another method is to place a stick upright under the center of the lean-to. This method, however, will restrict your space and movements in the shelter.

For additional protection from wind and rain, place some brush, your pack, or other equipment at the sides of the lean-to.

To reduce heat loss to the ground, place some type of insulating material, such as leaves or pine needles, inside your lean-to.

Note: When at rest, you lose as much as 80 percent of your body heat to the ground.

PONCHO TENT

This tent provides a low silhouette. It also protects you from the elements on two sides. It has, however, less usable space and observation area than a lean-to. To make this tent, you need a poncho, two 1.5-to 2.5-meter ropes, six sharpened sticks about 30 centimeters long, and two trees 2 to 3 meters apart.

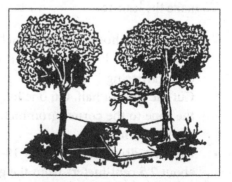

Poncho tent using overhanging branch.

To make the tent:

- Tie off the poncho hood in the same way as the poncho lean-to.
- Tie a 1.5-to 2.5-meter rope to the center grommet on each side of the poncho.
- Tie the other ends of these ropes at about knee height to two trees 2 to 3 meters apart and stretch the poncho tight.
- Draw one side of the poncho tight and secure it to the ground pushing sharpened sticks through the grommets.
- Follow the same procedure on the other side.

If you need a center support, use the same methods as for the poncho lean-to. Another center support is an A-frame set outside but over the center of the tent. Use two 90-to 120-centimeter-long sticks, one with a forked end, to form the A-frame. Tie the hood's drawstring to the A-frame to support the center of the tent.

FIELD-EXPEDIENT LEAN-TO

If you are in a wooded area and have enough natural materials, you can make a field-expedient lean-to without the aid of tools or with only a knife. It takes longer to make this type of shelter than it does to make other types, but it will protect you from the elements.

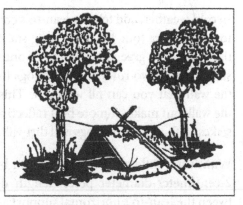

Poncho tent with A-frame.

You will need two trees (or upright poles) about 2 meters apart; one pole about 2 meters long and 2.5 centimeters in diameter; five to eight poles about 3 meters long and 2.5 centimeters in diameter for beams; cord or vines for securing the horizontal support to the trees; and other poles, saplings, or vines to crisscross the beams.

To make this lean-to:

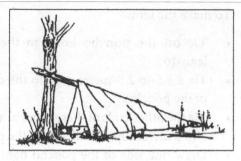

One-man shelter.

- Tie the 2-meter pole to the two trees at waist to chest height. This is the horizontal support. If a standing tree is not available, construct a biped using Y-shaped sticks or two tripods.
- Place one end of the beams (3-meter poles) on one side of the horizontal support. As with all lean-to type shelters, be sure to place the lean-to's backside into the wind.
- Crisscross saplings or vines on the beams.
- Cover the framework with brush, leaves, pine needles, or grass, starting at the bottom and working your way up like shingling.
- Place straw, leaves, pine needles, or grass inside the shelter for bedding.

In cold weather, add to your lean-to's comfort by building a fire reflector wall. Drive four 1.5-meter-long stakes into the ground to support the wall. Stack green logs on top of one another between the support stakes. Form two rows of stacked logs to create an inner space within the wall that you can fill with dirt. This action not only strengthens the wall, but makes it more heat reflective. Bind the top of the support stakes so that the green logs and dirt will stay in place.

With just a little more effort you can have a drying rack. Cut a few 2-centimeter-diameter poles (length depends on the distance between the lean-to's horizontal support and the top of the fire reflector wall). Lay one end of the poles on the lean-to support and the other end on top of the reflector wall. Place and tie into place smaller sticks across these poles. You now have a place to dry clothes, meat, or fish.

SWAMP BED

In a marsh or swamp, or any area with standing water or continually wet ground, the swamp bed keeps you out of the water.

When selecting such a site, consider the weather, wind, tides, and available materials. To make a swamp bed:

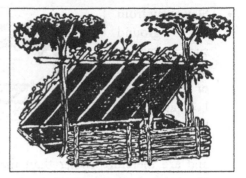

Field-expedient lean-to and fire reflector.

- Look for four trees clustered in a rectangle, or cut four poles (bamboo is ideal) and drive them firmly into the ground so they form a rectangle. They should be far enough apart and strong enough to support your height and weight, to include equipment.
- Cut two poles that span the width of the rectangle. They, too, must be strong enough to support your weight.
- Secure these two poles to the trees (or poles). Be sure they are high enough above the ground or water to allow for tides and high water.
- Cut additional poles that span the rectangle's length. Lay them across the two side poles, and secure them.
- Cover the top of the bed frame with broad leaves or grass to form a soft sleeping surface.
- Build a fire pad by laying clay, silt, or mud on one comer of the swamp bed and allow it to dry.

Another shelter designed to get you above and out of the water or wet ground uses the same rectangular configuration as the swamp bed. You very simply lay sticks and branches lengthwise on the inside of the trees (or poles) until there is enough material to raise the sleeping surface above the water level.

NATURAL SHELTERS
Do not overlook natural formations that provide shelter. Examples are caves, rocky crevices, clumps of bushes, small depressions, large rocks on leeward sides of hills, large trees with low-hanging limbs, and fallen trees with thick branches. However, when selecting a natural formation:

- Stay away from low ground such as ravines, narrow valleys, or creek beds. Low areas collect the heavy cold air at night

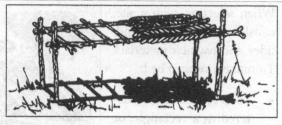

Swamp bed.

and are therefore colder than the surrounding high ground. Thick, brushy, low ground also harbors more insects.

- Check for poisonous snakes, ticks, mites, scorpions, and stinging ants.
- Look for loose rocks, dead limbs, coconuts, or other natural growth than could fall on your shelter.

DEBRIS HUT

For warmth and ease of construction, this shelter is one of the best. When shelter is essential to survival, build this shelter.

To make a debris hut:

- Build it by making a tripod with two short stakes and a long ridgepole or by placing one end of a long ridgepole on top of a sturdy base.

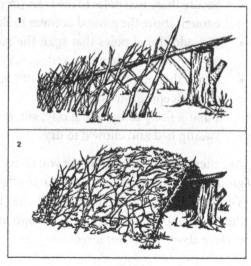

Debris hut.

- Secure the ridgepole (pole running the length of the shelter) using the tripod method or by anchoring it to a tree at about waist height.

- Prop large sticks along both sides of the ridgepole to create a wedge-shaped ribbing effect. Ensure the ribbing is wide enough to accommodate your body and steep enough to shed moisture.
- Place finer sticks and brush crosswise on the ribbing. These form a latticework that will keep the insulating material (grass, pine needles, leaves) from falling through the ribbing into the sleeping area.
- Add light, dry, if possible, soft debris over the ribbing until the insulating material is at least 1 meter thick—the thicker the better.
- Place a 30-centimeter layer of insulating material inside the shelter.
- At the entrance, pile insulating material that you can drag to you once inside the shelter to close the entrance or build a door.
- As a final step in constructing this shelter, add shingling material or branches on top of the debris layer to prevent the insulating material from blowing away in a storm.

TREE-PIT SNOW SHELTER

If you are in a cold, snow-covered area where evergreen trees grow and you have a digging tool, you can make a tree-pit shelter.

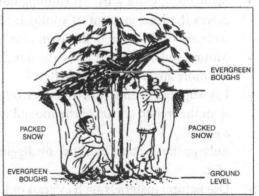

Tree-pit snow shelter.

To make this shelter:

- Find a tree with bushy branches that provides overhead cover.
- Dig out the snow around the tree trunk until you reach the depth and diameter you desire, or until you reach the ground.
- Pack the snow around the top and the inside of the hole to provide support.

- Find and cut other evergreen boughs. Place them over the top of the pit to give you additional overhead cover. Place evergreen boughs in the bottom of the pit for insulation.

BEACH SHADE SHELTER

This shelter protects you from the sun, wind, rain, and heat. It is easy to make using natural materials. To make this shelter:

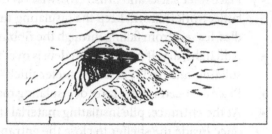

Beach shade shelter.

- Find and collect driftwood or other natural material to use as support beams and as a digging tool.
- Select a site that is above the high water mark.
- Scrape or dig out a trench running north to south so that it receives the least amount of sunlight. Make the trench long and wide enough for you to lie down comfortably.
- Mound soil on three sides of the trench. The higher the mound, the more space inside the shelter.
- Lay support beams (driftwood or other natural material) that span the trench on top of the mound to form the framework for a roof.
- Enlarge the shelter's entrance by digging out more sand in front of it.
- Use natural materials such as grass or leaves to form a bed inside the shelter.

DESERT SHELTERS

In an arid environment, consider the time, effort, and material needed to make a shelter. If you have material such as a poncho, or canvas, use it along with such terrain features as rock outcropping, mounds of sand, or a depression between dunes or rocks to make your shelter.

Using rock outcroppings:

- Anchor one end of your poncho (canvas or other material) on the edge of the outcrop using rocks or other weights.
- Extend and anchor the other end of the poncho so it provides the best possible shade.

In a sandy area:

- Build a mound of sand or use the side of a sand dune for one side of the shelter.
- Anchor one end of the material on top of the mound using sand or other weights.
- Extend and anchor the other end of the material so it provides the best possible shade.

Note: If you have enough material, fold it in half and form a 30-centimeter to 45-centimeter airspace between the two halves. This airspace will reduce the temperature under the shelter.

A belowground shelter can reduce the midday heat as much as 16 to 22 degrees C (30 to 40 degrees F). Building it, however, requires more time and effort than for other shelters. Since your physical effort will make you sweat more and increase dehydration, construct it before the heat of the day.

To make this shelter:

- Find a low spot or depression between dunes or rocks. If necessary, dig a trench 45 to 60 centimeters deep and long and wide enough for you to lie in comfortably.
- Pile the sand you take from the trench to form a mound around three sides.
- On the open end of the trench, dig out more sand so you can get in and out of your shelter easily.
- Cover the trench with your material.

• Secure the material in place using sand, rocks, or other weights.

If you have extra material, you can further decrease the midday temperature in the trench by securing the material 30 to 45 centimeters above the other cover. This layering of the material will reduce the inside temperature 11 to 22 degrees C (20 to 40 degrees F).

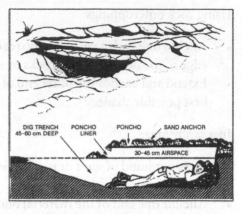

Belowground desert shelter.

Another type of belowground shade shelter is of similar construction, except all sides are open to air currents and circulation. For maximum protection, you need a minimum of two layers of parachute material. White is the best color to reflect heat; the innermost layer should be of darker material.

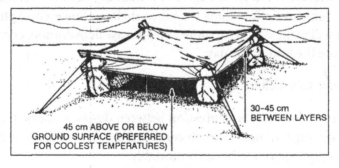

Open desert shelter.

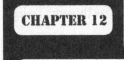

CHAPTER 12

PROJECT: HOW TO START A FIRE WITH A BATTERY

Being a DIY prepper involves learning multiple disciplines, and although I believe living off the land in a wilderness setting is an unrealistic TEOTWAWKI (The End Of The World As We Know It) plan, I still think everyone should have basic wilderness survival skills. One outdoor skill everyone should possess is the ability to make fire.

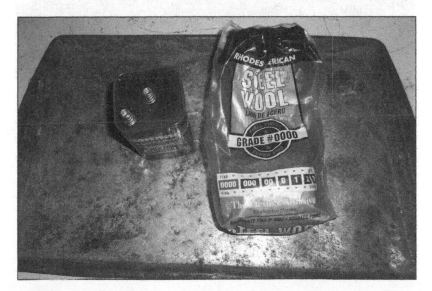

This is one skill in which redundancy is especially useful. Today's project involves using steel wool and a battery to light a fire. Once the basics are understood this process is repeatable with almost an unlimited variety of batteries. Theoretically, it can even be done using a remote control.

All you need to do is take a piece of fine steel wool—the finer the better (I use 0000 grade)—pull it apart a little to separate a few threads. To light

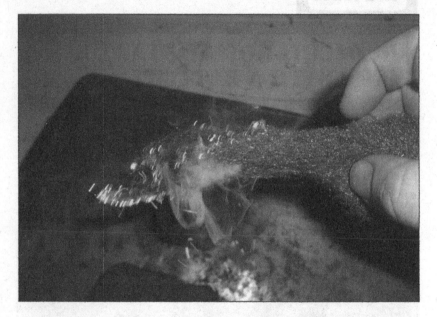

it, take the steel wool threads and short-circuit a battery by connecting the wool to both battery terminals. Be careful, because the steel will immediately turn red hot. Blow on it a little and it will burst into flame. You can make it even more effective by mixing in a little dryer lint.

Once you have lit a fire with a lantern battery or a 9-volt battery and seen how easy it is, you can take the back off a flashlight, turn it on and use the battery and the metal flashlight case to do the same thing. Once you understand the science behind it, you can readily adapt it to other types of batteries. I have even repeated this process using cell phone batteries.

CHAPTER 13

WATER PROCUREMENT

Water is one of your most urgent needs in a survival situation. You can't live long without it, especially in hot areas where you lose water rapidly through perspiration. Even in cold areas, you need a minimum of 2 liters of water each day to maintain efficiency.

More than three-fourths of your body is composed of fluids. Your body loses fluid as a result of heat, cold, stress, and exertion. To function effectively, you must replace the fluid your body loses. So, one of your first goals is to obtain an adequate supply of water.

WATER SOURCES

Almost any environment has water present to some degree. The graph starting on page 66 lists possible sources of water in various environments. It also provides information on how to make the water potable.

Note: If you do not have a canteen, a cup, a can, or other type of container, improvise one from plastic or water-resistant cloth. Shape the plastic or cloth into a bowl by pleating it. Use pins or other suitable items—even your hands—to hold the pleats.

Envi-ronment	Source of Water	Means of Obtaining and/or Making Potable	Remarks
Frigid areas	Snow and ice	Melt and purify.	**Do not eat** without melting! Eating snow and ice can reduce body temperature and will lead to more dehydrating. Snow and ice are no purer than the water from which they come. Sea ice that is gray in color or opaque is salty. Do not use it without desalting it. Sea ice that is crystalline with a bluish cast has little salt in it.
At sea	Sea	Use desalter kit if available.	**Do not** drink seawater without desalting.
	Rain	Catch rain in tarps or in other water-holding material or containers.	If tarp or water-holding material has become encrusted with salt, wash it in the sea before using (very little salt will remain on it).
	Sea ice		See remarks above for frigid areas.
Beach	Ground	Dig hole deep enough to allow water to seep in; obtain rocks, build fire, and heat rocks; drop hot rocks in water; hold cloth over hole to absorb steam; wring water from cloth.	Alternate method if a container or bark pot is available: Fill container or pot with seawater; build fire and boil water to produce steam; hold cloth over container to absorb steam; wring water from cloth.

Environment	Source of Water	Means of Obtaining and/or Making Potable	Remarks
Desert	Ground • in valleys and low areas • at foot of concave bands of dry river beads • at foot of cliffs or rock outcrops • at first depression behind first sand dune of dry desert lakes • wherever you find damp surface sand • wherever you find green vegetation	Dig holes deep enough to allow water to seep in.	In a sand dune belt, any available water will be found beneath the original valley floor at the edge of dunes.
	Cacti	Cut off the top of a barrel cactus and mash or squeeze the pulp. **CAUTION: Do not eat pulp. Place pulp in mouth, suck out juice, and discard pulp.**	Without a machete, cutting into a cactus is difficult and takes time since you must get past the long, strong spines and cut through the tough rind.
	Depressions or holes in rocks		Periodic rainfall may collect in pools, seep into fissures, or collect in holes in rocks
	Fissures in rocks	Insert flexible tubing and siphon water. If fissure is large enough, you can lower a container into it.	

67

Environment	Source of Water	Means of Obtaining and/or Making Potable	Remarks
	Porous rock	Insert flexible tubing and siphon water.	
	Condensation on metal	Use cloth to absorb water, then wring water from cloth.	Extreme temperature variations between night and day may cause condensation on metal surfaces. Following are signs to water for in the desert to help you find water: All trails lead to water. You should follow in the direction in which the trails converge. Signs of camps, campfire ashes, animal droppings, and trampled terrain may mark trails. Flocks of birds will circle over water holes. Some birds fly to water holes at dawn and sunset. Their flight at these times is generally fast and close to the ground. Bird tracks or chirping sounds in the evening or early morning sometimes indicate that water is nearby.

Water sources in different environments.

If you do not have a reliable source to replenish your water supply, stay alert for ways in which your environment can help you.

Heavy dew can provide water. Tie rags or tufts of fine grass around your ankles and walk through dew-covered grass before sunrise. As the rags or grass tufts absorb the dew, wring the water into a container. Repeat the process until you have a supply of water or until the dew is gone. Australian natives sometimes mop up as much as a liter an hour this way.

Bees or ants going into a hole in a tree may point to a water-filled hole. Siphon the water with plastic tubing or scoop it up with an improvised dipper. You can also stuff cloth in the hole to absorb the water and then wring it from the cloth.

Water sometimes gathers in tree crotches or rock crevices. Use the above procedures to get the water. In arid areas, bird droppings around a crack in the rocks may indicate water in or near the crack.

Green bamboo thickets are an excellent source of fresh water. Water from green bamboo is clear and odorless. To get the water, bend a green bamboo stalk, tie it down, and cut off the top. The water will drip freely during the night. Old, cracked bamboo may contain water.

Fluid	Remarks
Alcoholic beverages	Dehydrate the body and cloud judgment.
Urine	Contains harmful body wastes. Is about 2 percent salt.
Blood	Is salty and considered a food; therefore, requires additional body fluids to digest. May transmit disease.
Seawater	Is about 4 percent salt. It takes about 2 liters of body fluids to rid the body of waste from 1 liter of seawater. Therefore, by drinking seawater you deplete your body's water supply, which can cause death.

The effects of substitute fluids.

CAUTION
Purify the water before drinking it.

In tropical areas, wherever you find banana or plantain trees, you can get water. Cut down the tree, leaving about a 30-centimeter stump, and scoop out the center of the stump so that the hollow is bowl-shaped. Water from the roots will immediately start to fill the hollow. The first three fillings of water will be bitter, but succeeding fillings will be palatable. The stump will supply water for up to four days. Be sure to cover it to keep out insects.

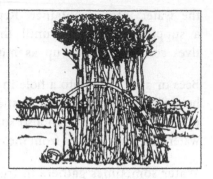

Water from green bamboo.

Some tropical vines can give you water. Cut a notch in the vine as high as you can reach, then cut the vine off close to the ground. Catch the dropping liquid in a container or in your mouth (Figure 6-5).

> **CAUTION**
> Do not drink the liquid if it is sticky, milky, or bitter tasting.

The milk from green (unripe) coconuts is a good thirst quencher. However, the milk from mature coconuts contains an oil that acts as a laxative. Drink in moderation only.

In the American tropics you may find large trees whose branches support air plants. These air plants may hold a considerable amount of rainwater in their overlapping, thickly growing leaves. Strain the water through a cloth to remove insects and debris.

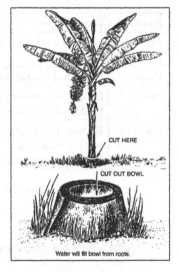

CUT HERE

CUT OUT BOWL

Water will fill bowl from roots.

You can get water from plants with moist pulpy centers. Cut off a section of the plant and squeeze or smash the pulp so that the moisture runs out. Catch the liquid in a container.

Water from plantain or banana tree stump.

Plant roots may provide water. Dig or pry the roots out of the ground, cut them into short pieces, and smash the pulp so that the moisture runs out. Catch the liquid in a container.

Fleshy leaves, stems, or stalks, such as bamboo, contain water. Cut or notch the stalks at the base of a joint to drain out the liquid.

The following trees can also provide water:

- *Palms.* Palms, such as the buri, coconut, sugar, rattan, and nips, contain liquid. Bruise a lower frond and pull it down so the tree will "bleed" at the injury.
- *Traveler's tree.* Found in Madagascar, this tree has a cuplike sheath at the base of its leaves in which water collects.
- *Umbrella tree.* The leaf bases and roots of this tree of western tropical Africa can provide water.
- *Baobab tree.* This tree of the sandy plains of northern Australia and Africa collects water in its bottlelike trunk during the wet season. Frequently, you can find clear, fresh water in these trees after weeks of dry weather.

Water from a vine.

> **CAUTION**
> Do not keep the sap from plants longer than 24 hours. It begins fermenting, becoming dangerous as a water source.

STILL CONSTRUCTION

You can use stills in various areas of the world. They draw moisture from the ground and from plant material. You need certain materials to build a still, and you need time to let it collect the water. It takes about 24 hours to get 0.5 to 1 liter of water.

ABOVEGROUND STILL

To make the aboveground still, you need a sunny slope on which to place the still, a clear plastic bag, green leafy vegetation, and a small rock.

To make the still:

- Fill the bag with air by turning the opening into the breeze or by "scooping" air into the bag.
- Fill the plastic bag half to three-fourths full of green leafy vegetation.
- Be sure to remove all hard sticks or sharp spines that might puncture the bag.

CAUTION
Do not use poisonous vegetation. It will provide poisonous liquid.

- Place a small rock or similar item in the bag.
- Close the bag and tie the mouth securely as close to the end of the bag as possible to keep the maximum amount of air space. If you have a piece of tubing, a small straw, or a hollow reed, insert one end in the mouth of the bag before you tie it securely. Then tie off or plug the tubing so that air will not escape. This tubing will allow you to drain out condensed water without untying the bag.
- Place the bag, mouth downhill, on a slope in full sunlight. Position the mouth of the bag slightly higher than the low point in the bag.
- Settle the bag in place so that the rock works itself into the low point in the bag.

To get the condensed water from the still, loosen the tie around the bag's mouth and tip the bag so that the water collected around the rock will drain out. Then retie the mouth securely and reposition the still to allow further condensation.

Change the vegetation in the bag after extracting most of the water from it. This will ensure maximum output of water.

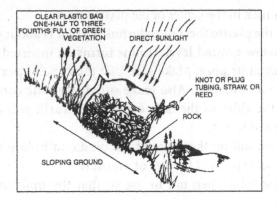

CLEAR PLASTIC BAG
ONE-HALF TO THREE-
FOURTHS FULL OF GREEN
VEGETATION

DIRECT SUNLIGHT

KNOT OR PLUG
TUBING, STRAW, OR
REED

ROCK

SLOPING GROUND

Aboveground solar water still.

BELOWGROUND STILL

To make a belowground still, you need a digging tool, a container, a clear plastic sheet, a drinking tube, and a rock.

Select a site where you believe the soil will contain moisture (such as a dry stream bed or a low spot where rainwater has collected). The soil at this site should be easy to dig, and sunlight must hit the site most of the day.

To construct the still:

- Dig a bowl-shaped hole about 1 meter across and 60 centimeters deep.
- Dig a sump in the center of the hole. The sump's depth and perimeter will depend on the size of the container that you have to place in it. The bottom of the sump should allow the container to stand upright.
- Anchor the tubing to the container's bottom by forming a loose overhand knot in the tubing.
- Place the container upright in the sump.
- Extend the unanchored end of the tubing up, over, and beyond the lip of the hole.
- Place the plastic sheet over the hole, covering its edges with soil to hold it in place.

- Place a rock in the center of the plastic sheet.
- Lower the plastic sheet into the hole until it is about 40 centimeters below ground level. It now forms an inverted cone with the rock at its apex. Make sure that the cone's apex is directly over your container. Also make sure the plastic cone does not touch the sides of the hole because the earth will absorb the condensed water.
- Put more soil on the edges of the plastic to hold it securely in place and to prevent the loss of moisture.
- Plug the tube when not in use so that the moisture will not evaporate.

You can drink water without disturbing the still by using the tube as a straw.

You may want to use plants in the hole as a moisture source. If so, dig out additional soil from the sides of the hole to form a slope on which to place the plants. Then proceed as above.

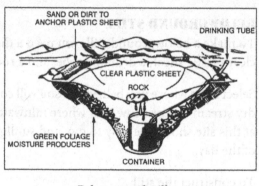

Belowground still.

If polluted water is your only moisture source, dig a small trough outside the hole about 25 centimeters from the still's lip. Dig the trough about 25 centimeters deep and 8 centimeters wide. Pour the polluted water in the trough. Be sure you do not spill any polluted water around the rim of the hole where the plastic sheet touches the soil. The trough holds the polluted water and the soil filters it as the still draws it. The water then condenses on the plastic and drains into the container. This process works extremely well when your only water source is salt water.

You will need at least three stills to meet your individual daily water intake needs.

WATER PURIFICATION

Rainwater collected in clean containers or in plants is usually safe for drinking. However, purify water from lakes, ponds, swamps, springs, or streams, especially the water near human settlements or in the tropics. When possible, purify all water you got from vegetation or from the ground by using iodine or chlorine, or by boiling.

Traditional methods of purifying water are:

- Using water purification tablets. (Follow the directions provided.)
- Placing 5 drops of 2 percent tincture of iodine in a canteen full of clear water. If the canteen is full of cloudy or cold water, use 10 drops. (Let the canteen of water stand for 30 minutes before drinking.)
- Boiling water for 1 minute at sea level, adding 1 minute for each additional 300 meters above sea level, or boil for 10 minutes no matter where you are.

While these methods are effective, small portable and reusable filtration devices are now readily available and come in various sizes and weights. These devices can filter gallons of water and can effectively screen waterborne pathogens down to 2 microns, providing a safe source of potable water.

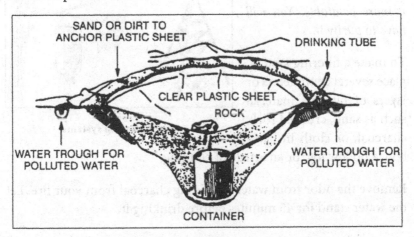

Belowground still to get potable water from polluted water.

By drinking nonpotable water you may contract diseases or swallow organisms that can harm you. Examples of such diseases or organisms are:

- *Dysentery.* Severe, prolonged diarrhea with bloody stools, fever, and weakness.
- *Cholera and typhoid.* You may be susceptible to these diseases regardless of inoculations.
- *Flukes.* Stagnant, polluted water—especially in tropical areas—often contains blood flukes. If you swallow flukes, they will bore into the bloodstream, live as parasites, and cause disease.
- *Leeches.* If you swallow a leech, it can hook onto the throat passage or inside the nose. It will suck blood, create a wound, and move to another area. Each bleeding wound may become infected.

WATER FILTRATION DEVICES

If the water you find is also muddy, stagnant, and foul smelling, and you do not have a portable filtration device, you can clear the water:

- By placing it in a container and letting it stand for 12 hours.
- By pouring it through a filtering system.

Note: These procedures only clear the water and make it more palatable. You will have to purify it.

To make a filtering system, place several centimeters or layers of filtering material such as sand, crushed rock, charcoal, or cloth in bamboo, a hollow log, or an article of clothing.

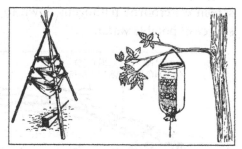

Water filtering systems.

Remove the odor from water by adding charcoal from your fire. Let the water stand for 45 minutes before drinking it.

CHAPTER 14

FILL YOUR PANTRY

A long-term food storage plan is your very own "food bank account."
You want that bank account to be a sound investment, one that you
have ready access to, and one that will provide you exactly what you
need when you need it. Remember: no matter what a great deal it is,
how long its shelf life, or how practical it might sound, there is abso-
lutely no point in storing food you don't want to eat.

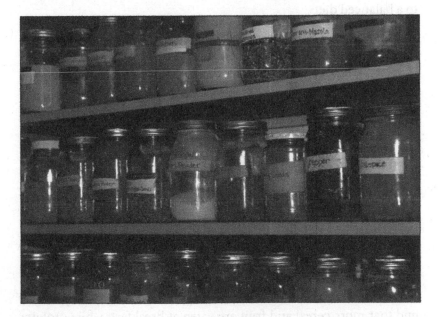

SO WHAT SHOULD GO INTO YOUR FOOD PANTRY?

Build your own individualized food pantry using the common-sense "eat what you store, store what you eat" approach. This means that you only buy food you actually want to eat, food that your family is accustomed to, and food that you actually use every day, rather than accumulating food and locking it up tight for some future imagined time.

Because you are always rotating through your pantry, you don't have to wait for a full-scale emergency to use your food. You always have your own piggy bank to draw from, even when it's just a week where your budget is a little pinched.

To start creating your own customized food pantry, consider the kinds of meals your family currently eats. Look at your favorite recipes and see how you might adapt those to items that are in a storage pantry. Try to take a balanced approach to meal planning and storage. The following ratios are an example of foods that would contribute to a balanced diet:

PROTEIN: 13 percent of your food supply. This category includes legumes, meat, peanut butter, and assorted nuts.

GRAINS: 40 percent of your food supply. This would include cereals like oatmeal, as well as pasta, rice, and breads.

VEGETABLES: 20 percent of your food supply. This would include carrots, peas, green beans, corn, and other vegetables.

DAIRY: 12 percent of your food supply. This would include milk, yogurt, and cheeses.

FRUITS: 15 percent of your food supply. This would include canned peaches, berries, and other fruits, including tomatoes.

These ratios are only a guideline and apply to a full day, so you may find that more cereal and fruit are eaten at breakfast, while proteins and vegetables make up the rest of the day's meals.

STAPLES

Your long-term food storage plan begins with the fundamentals, including grains, beans, fats, sweeteners, dairy items, and basic baking ingredients.

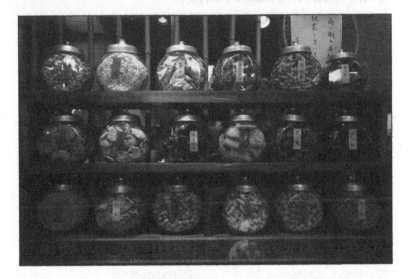

At the most basic level, every person needs about one pound of dry matter every day to survive. Dry matter may mean legumes, grains, sugar, pasta, dried vegetables, or rice. This dry matter represents calories, the stuff that is needed to produce energy in the body. A pound of dry matter represents about 1,600 calories, a reasonable amount of energy for the average adult. A consistent diet of dry matter would, of course, be deadly dull, and over the course of a few months, the body would begin to suffer from the lack of protein, fresh greens, and essential vitamins. Still, it is good to keep in mind as you make decisions about what to store.

Some people do keep an emergency pantry that contains only these essentials—whole grains, dried beans, oils, and sweeteners. The problem is that these foods require that you to cook in a way that may not be compatible with your current lifestyle. You need to have a basic understanding of cooking and baking techniques, as well as a high tolerance for boring meals! If you decide to make these staples the center of your food pantry, take the time to learn to use them in your everyday meals.

A ONE-YEAR EMERGENCY PANTRY

To feed a family of four for a full year, a pantry that consisted entirely of staple ingredients would look something like this:

500 pounds of whole grain wheat for grinding
100 pounds of flour
100 pounds of cornmeal
100 pounds of oats
50 pounds of quinoa
50 pounds of millet
200 pounds of rice
100 pounds of pasta
120 pounds of dried beans
20 pounds of lentils
20 pounds of split peas
40 pounds of soy beans
16 pounds of peanut butter
1½ gallons of dehydrated eggs
50 pounds of TVP

160 pounds of sugar
12 pounds of honey
12 pounds of molasses or maple syrup
12 pounds of jam
12 pounds of sprouting seeds
40 quarts of vegetable oil
240 pounds of dry milk
48 cans of evaporated milk
4 pounds of baking powder
4 pounds of baking soda
2 pounds of yeast
20 pounds of salt
2 gallons of vinegar
20 pounds of dry soup mix
A of spices and seasonings

LONG-TERM FOOD STORAGE

Every item in your storage pantry wants three conditions to maintain its optimum quality: cool, dry, and dark. High temperatures, humid or wet conditions, and exposure to light are the primary causes of spoiled food. In addition, food must be kept safe from bugs and rodents. Keep these factors in mind when storing any food products. The following are specific recommendations for each food group.

Whole grains, dried beans, and white rice are very durable, but they prefer to be stored in a cool, dry location. Flours, sugars, oils, dry milk, and canned goods want the same conditions, but generally have a shorter shelf life, so check on life expectancy before deciding on how much to store. Temperatures of 50–60°F are ideal for ensuring maximum longevity. Overheating or wide temperature swings will shorten shelf life. Likewise, humidity causes challenges. Any time moisture is present there is a danger for molds and bacteria to grow.

SHELF LIFE OF FOODS

"Sealed" refers to hermetically sealed containers. These are estimates, and will vary based on storage conditions. Check the manufacturer's dates for specific information.
For commercial products, check the manufacturer's "best by" date, and use that as your "sealed" date.

PROTEINS	SEALED	OPEN
Canned ham	2-5 years	3-4 days in refrigerator
Freeze-dried meats	25 years	1 year
Commercially made jerky	2 years	1 year
Home-dried jerky	1-2 months	1-2 months
Hard/dry sausage	6 weeks in pantry	3 weeks in refrigerator
Dried eggs	12-15 months	Refrigerate after opening. Use within 7 to 10 days. Use reconstituted egg mix immediately or refrigerate and use within 1 hour.
Canned tuna	18 months	3-4 days in refrigerator
Other canned meats	18 months	3-4 days in refrigerator
LEGUMES	**SEALED**	**OPEN**
Dried beans	30 years	5 years
Instant dried beans	30 years	1 year
TVP	10 years	1 year
Peanuts		
Peanut butter, natural	2 years from manufacturer's date	2-3 months
Peanut butter, emulsified	2 years from manufacturer's date	18 months
Peanut butter powder	4 years	1 year

Continued

GRAINS AND FLOUR

Wheat	10-12 years	2 years
Dry corn	10-12 years	3 years
Millet	10-12 years	4 years
Flax	10-12 years	4 years
Barley	8 years	18 months
Quinoa	20 years	1 year
Rolled oats	8 years	1 year
Whole wheat flour	2 years	6 months
White flour	4 years	1 year
Spelt flour	5 years	8-12 months
Flaxseed flour	1 year	2-3 months
White rice	10 years	1 year
Brown and wild rice	1-2 years	6 months
Pasta	8 years	3 years

NUTS	SEALED	OPEN
In the shell	9 months	6 months
Shelled	2 years	18 months

FRUITS AND VEGETABLES

Low-acid canned goods, such as soups, vegetables, stews	2-5 years	3-4 days in refrigerator
High-acid canned goods, such as fruits, tomatoes, and vinegar-based items	12-18 months	5-7 days in refrigerator
Home-canned foods	1 year	3-4 days in refrigerator
Dehydrated fruit	25 years	12-18 months
Dehydrated vegetables	25 years	1-2 years

BAKING SUPPLIES

Yeast	2 years	4 months
Honey	10 years	2 years
White sugar	30 years	2 years
Brown sugar	10 years	1 year

Molasses	2 years	6 months
Baking powder, baking soda, and salt	30 years	2 years
Vinegar	2 years	1 year
Spices and seasonings	2 years	2 years
Boullion	5 years	2 years
OILS	**SEALED**	**OPEN**
Cooking oils	6 months	3-6 months
Shortening	2 years from manufactured date	1 year
Shortening powder	10 years	1 year
DAIRY PRODUCTS		
Dry milk	25 years	2 years
Sour cream powder	10 years	1 year
Cheese, dried	15 years	6 months
Butter powder	5 years	9 months
OTHER		
Seeds for sprouting	5 years	4 years

All bulk foods used for long-term storage should be carefully sealed to keep them safe from pests and rodents. To store a large quantity of dried bulk foods, choose food-grade five-gallon buckets with gasket lids. Line each bucket with a Mylar bag. Place one 500cc oxygen absorber in the bottom of the bag. Fill the bag about half way, shaking the bucket to settle the food. Add another oxygen absorber, and then fill the bucket, leaving about an inch of space on top. Place another oxygen absorber on top.

Pull the bag up as high as you can, settling the food into the bucket. Use a hot iron to seal the Mylar bag. Place a board on the edge of the bucket, lay the bag top straight and start sealing the bag from left to right, making sure to squeeze out excess air before finishing the seal. Fold the bag down, and place the gasket lid on the bucket.

USING OXYGEN ABSORBERS

Oxygen absorbers begin absorbing oxygen the moment they are exposed to air, so don't open your package until you are ready to use them. Remove only the number you need, and immediately place the remaining absorbers in a glass jar with a tight lid.

ROTATION

The "Store What You Eat and Eat What You Store" family pantry is a living, breathing organism. It is designed to use every day, not just in an emergency. Because, for the most part, you are stockpiling foods that are a standard part of your family's diet, you should have an easy time keeping foods fresh and used before their expiration dates.

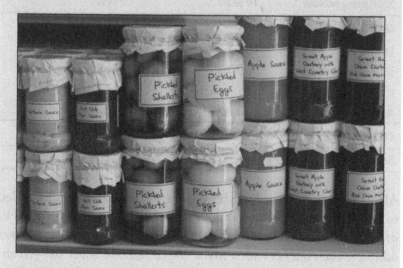

Always remember FIFO—first in, first out. Develop a system. You can keep older items front and center on your shelf, and fill your shelves from the rear when you add new foods. Or you can store from left to right, always using from the left and adding on the right. Food rotation shelving helps you create an almost foolproof system for your canned goods, feeding them to you in the order you fed them into the shelf.

CHAPTER 15

POWER AND LIGHT

Storms and technological failures often take out our power. In a major disaster power could be lost for a week or more. When the power goes off, the heater blower stops running. The refrigerator stops. The freezer thaws. The ATM won't work. Electric pumps at the gas station won't work. Folks in rural areas lose the pumps that supply their water. People with medical conditions can face life-or-death situations waiting for lifesaving gadgets to kick back on. Worse, the TV goes off right in the middle of that lame reality show.

Of course, you can avoid these problems by investing in an emergency backup power system or by making arrangements with your rich neighbor to plug into his. Most of us will want our own. Since most of our appliances run on 120 volts AC, we basically have two options:

1. Buy a fuel-powered generator, or . . .
2. Use your car battery or a deep-cycle battery to power an inverter. An inverter is a device that changes 12-volt direct current from a battery into 120-volt AC.

The first step is to decide what you actually need and what you can afford. If you want to power a few fluorescent or LED lights, an electric blanket, and an emergency radio, you can get away with the inverter idea. If you want to keep your refrigerator going and run an electric heater and have plenty of light, you'll need a generator.

Electrical power is measured in watts. All appliances have an operating power. Devices that employ electrical motors or other devices that need an electrical kick also have what's called a *surge wattage*, which means extra watts are required to start the motor or device.

Common appliances and their typical power requirements	
Blow Dryer	900–1500 watts
CD/DVD player	35 watts
Clock radio	30–100 watts
Common light bulb	60 watts
Fan	75 watts (150 watts surge)
Color TV	300 watts (400 watts surge)
Coffee maker	650–1200 watts
Desktop computer system	400 watts (600 watts surge)
Electric blanket	80–100 watts
Electric heating pad	12–36 watts
Game box	100 watts
Microwave oven	750 watts (1500 watts surge)
Iron	1000 watts
Toaster	800–1500 watts
Furnace fan	750 watts (1500 watts surge)
Refrigerator	600–1200 watts (1200–2400 watts surge)
Vacuum cleaner	300–1100 watts
Satellite receiver	30 watts
Space heater	300–1100 watts
Stereo	30–100 watts
Washing machine	950 watts
Water cooler	120 watts
Well pump	2,400 watts (3,600 watts surge)
Electric water heater	4,500 watts
Whole-house AC or heat pump	15,000 watts (30,000 watts surge)

To figure out your power needs, add up the normal wattage figures for all the devices you might be using at the same time. Take the figures from this list or directly off the manufacturer's service tag on the device. If it doesn't give the wattage it will likely give the volts and amps. Multiply volts and amps together to get the watts. Add 20 percent to account for surge wattage. If a generator can't handle the surge wattage, the start up power will be unstable and can damage TVs and computers. Also, switching on a big-power device can cause the power to falter. Protect electronic devices with a good surge protector and/or an uninterruptible power supply (UPS).

Plan to stagger usage as much as possible. If you ensure your devices will not all be turned on at the same time, you can get along with a smaller, less expensive generator, or possibly even an inverter.

1. GENERATORS

Generators today are relatively cheap and are an easy way to get backup power. For instance, a reliable Coleman generator that produces 2500 watts and over 3100 surge can be purchased for under $500 and will provide 10 hours of power on a 3 gallon tank of gas. Propane-and diesel-burning generators are also available. When the diesel fuel is gone, diesel generators can burn filtered vegetable oils or an oil and diesel mix, but it will eventually clog the fuel injectors.

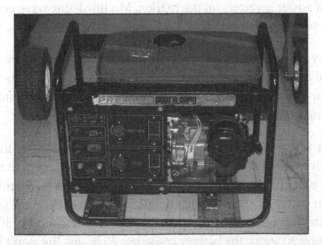

For long-term backup power a heavy-duty generator will outlast a light recreational generator, and a larger fuel tank like this one will let the generator run longer before refueling is required.

Generators do have some distinct disadvantages. They produce toxic fumes and must be run outside away from windows and doors. They tend to break down frequently. They make a lot of noise (some are far better than others in that regard). And they require large quantities of fuel, which must be stored somewhere where it won't be a hazard. Gasoline has a short shelf-life, even with stabilizers added. I have used gasoline that was stored for over a year without chemical stabilizers. Fuel storage should be rotated on a frequent basis.

2. INVERTERS

Using an inverter for emergency power is an excellent choice if your power needs are limited. Inverters are devices that change 12-volt battery power to 120-volt AC power. There are two general types of power inverters: true-sine wave and modified-sine wave (square wave). True-sine wave inverters produce power that is either identical to or sometimes slightly better than power from the power company. The power wave when viewed through an oscilloscope is a smooth sine wave.

Modified-sine wave and square wave inverters are the most common types of power inverters on the market. Modified-sine wave power inverters produce a power wave that is sufficient for most devices.

Before you purchase an inverter you will want to take a piece of paper and a pen and write down all of the appliances that you feel are necessary to have during a power outage, *then figure out their total operating wattage.*

Smaller watt totals (say, under 300 watts) can get along with an inexpensive small inverter that costs under $50. Inverters in that range can be plugged directly into the car's lighter socket. Depending on your car battery's reserve capacity rating, a good battery will give you 150 watts for an hour or two without the engine running. If you're only using 20 watts, the battery could last 20 hours. But don't let it go that far. Run the engine often to recharge the battery. To run a larger inverter (over 300 watts), you'll want to connect it directly to the car's battery with the cables provided, and you will need to run the engine continuously. A car's alternator can only supply about 700 watts maximum. It's best to purchase an inverter well under that wattage if you don't want to start blowing car fuses. However, if more power is needed, it's feasible to run inverters of 1,750 watts or more off of multiple batteries in parallel or deep-cycle batteries (these are different from your car battery). But at that point it would probably be just as cheap and easier to buy a generator.

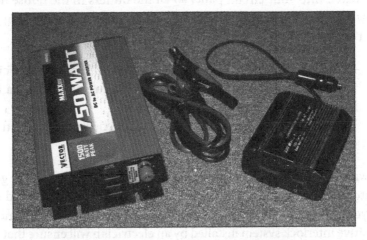

Left: a 750 watt (1500 peak watt) inverter that clamps to battery posts. Right: a 150 watt (300 peak watt) inverter that plugs into a car lighter socket.

When you hook a big inverter up to your vehicle battery, you will want to try to keep the inverter close to the battery, and out of the rain or snow.

It makes sense to have both generator and inverter backup capabilities. They can be staggered to provide different wattages at peak and low usage periods.

3. HOW TO WIRE YOUR HOUSE OR BUILDING

The easiest way by far to bring electricity in from the generator or inverter is to run in extension cords. You can run cords in for individual appliances, or you can run in a cord with multiple outlets.

The disadvantage to multiple outlets is that you will have to closely police them so the group is not plugging in at the wrong time and overloading the system.

If you have super-high wattage or voltage requirements (for instance, if you want to run your furnace blower or a well pump) or are dependent on 240-volts for major appliances, you're going to need a big expensive generator, and you'll want to consider having the generator wired into your circuit panel so all the outlets in the house have power. If you decide to do that, you must understand several important things:

- Do not try to wire the panel yourself unless you are an electrician. You've spent gobs of money on that big generator, spend a few more dollars on proper installation.
- Be sure to have the generator grounded according to the instructions in the operator's manual.

Always cut your house off from the power grid before starting the generator. If you don't, your precious electricity will be transmitted out of your home and it could electrocute anyone working on the line. A positive interlock system installed by an electrician will ensure that the house main breaker is cut off when the generator's breaker turns on.

4. OTHER SYSTEMS

Any system that supplies the needs of an entire home or building is going to cost a lot of money to construct. Solar, wind, and water systems are extremely expensive to build and only work when it's sunny, windy, or the water's flowing. If you're going to rely on solar systems for large power needs, you're going to need several hundred watts of solar power to keep the batteries charged, or run a generator to do it. The big concern with complicated systems is this: if you don't take care of it, it will not work when you need it and you will have wasted your money.

If you don't know anything about electricity, don't try installing electrical systems of any kind. You can burn down your house, fry your car, electrocute your children and the repairman, cause an explosion, cause battery acid burns and toxic gas exposures, and fibrillate your own heart. Be sensible.

5. IN THE EVENT OF A BLACKOUT

- Before you rig up your alternative power sources, turn off or unplug all devices to avoid a damaging surge when the power comes back on.
- Maintain your refrigerator/freezer protocol
- If appliances get wet, turn of the power main, unplug the appliances, and allow them to dry out before plugging them in again.

GENERATOR SAFETY

Take the following precautions when using a generator:

- Don't plug your generator into a regular household outlet. You can kill somebody outside your building and not even know it.
- Don't overload the generator. Add up the watts of your appliances and leave some room for surge voltages.
- Don't use a generator indoors or in an attached garage. Place it where carbon monoxide will not drift into your building. Operate it outdoors in a well ventilated area away from windows and airvents and protected from the weather.
- Use proper power cords that are heavy duty and rated for use outdoors. Cords are a trip hazard. Tape them in place, but do not put them under the carpet where they can overheat.
- Make sure your generator is properly grounded, according to the instructions in the operator's manual.
- Do not store fuel indoors
- Do not refuel while the generator is still running or when it is still hot.
- All equipment powered by the generator should be tunred off before shutting the generator down.
- The generator will get hot. Don't get burned.
- Keep children away from the generator.

BATTERIES
Some battery basics:

- For convenience, all your battery operated appliances and equipment should use the same battery size.
- Replaced stored batteries annually. If batteries are stored in a dry place at room temperature—not in a refrigerator or freezer—their shelf life can be as long as three years or more.
- Stick to disposable alkaline batteries or to rechargeable NiMH batteries. Lithium batteries are expensive. Alkaline batteries are cheaper than lithium, but lithium batteries work better at colder temperatures. NiCad batteries have two-thirds the life of alkaline batteries and can be recharged 500 times. Rechargeable NiMH batteries have four-fifths the life of alkaline batteries. You can get rechargeable alkaline batteries, but they have only half the life of disposable alkalines and they can only be recharged about 25 times.
- Chargers can be run off a generator, an inverter, and solar panels.
- If you are not going to use your flashlight or other device, remove the batteries to prevent damage from leaking battery acid.

6. ALTERNATE LIGHT SOURCES
Oil lamps, candles, kerosene lamps, and mantle lamps: Avoid them. They're a fire hazard. Kerosene oil lamps provide some limited heat as well as light. They're brighter than a candle but usually barely bright enough to read by. FYI, "lamp oil" is #1-grade kerosene.

If you're using these lamps, you must ventilate. Keep extra wicks in your disaster kit. Be careful where you place a lit lamp. It can get extremely hot above the lamp chimney. Glass can shatter. Metal-frame lamps are safer than glass-frame lamps.

Mantles are very fragile when ignited and require frequent replacement. The light of a mantle lamp is intense. Liquid fuel (white gas) requires pumping to pressurize the tank. Do not use unleaded gasoline in these lamps, unless the lantern is designed for it. Otherwise, the additives in the fuel will cause clogging.

Camp lamps with screw-in propane cannisters are the most conven-
ient of these types of lamps. There's no pumping and no spilling. Their
disadvantage is the fire hazard and the fact that they are less efficient
at cold temperatures.

Light sticks: These provide cool low-level light for several hours. The
light is non-directional, but can be rigged with a foil reflector to function as a flashlight.

Flashlights and headlamps: The normal iridescent bulbs that used to
be in all our flashlights waste most of their energy as heat. Fluorescent and LED lights are far more power-efficient. LED bulbs last over
10,000 hours and are shock and cold-resistant. Fluorescent bulbs last
ten times longer than iridescent bulbs but are not bright at cold temperatures. LED flashlights using groups of three to nine bulbs will
work six times as long as their equivalent iridescent bulbs on the
same batteries. LED lights now come in a big assortment of flashlights and headlights, using batteries, cranks, or solar power. Multi-
LED touchlamps for your home or car cost around $10.

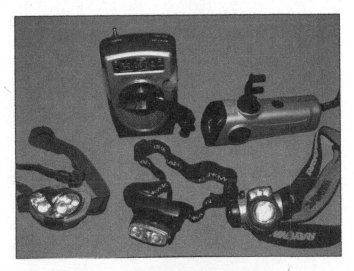

LED headlamps, flashlights, lamps.

CHAPTER 16

PROJECT: SUMAC LEMONADE

This project is a "wilderness survival" project. We are going to take staghorn sumac and make a refreshing drink often called "sumac-ade." Sumacs grow throughout the world, with staghorn sumac (*Rhus hirta* or *Rhus glabra*) being the most common type.

Although we don't use it as a spice here in North America, sumac "stags" are used as a traditional spice in many cultures in the Middle East. If you dry and grind staghorn sumac you will find it has a tangy flavor that is often used with grilled meats and fish.

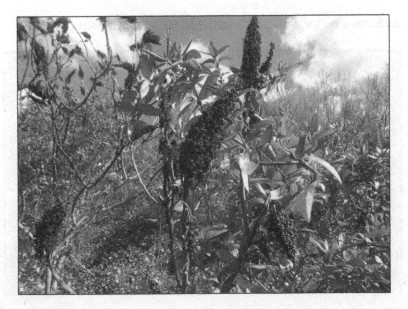

Though one should not eat wild food without first consulting a pictorial guide or an expert, it is very easy to distinguish staghorn sumac from poison sumac. The color of the berries is the biggest distinguisher.

Poison sumac has large white berries and only grows in wet areas—it is pretty rare.

Staghorn sumac has small red berries and is found all along country (and not so country) roads. I would bet that unless you live in a huge metropolis, you have seen sumac growing along the road.

Besides being a very cheap drink that tastes a lot like pink lemonade at a *fraction* of the cost, it has some health benefits, too. It is a good source of ascorbic acid—so preppers can use it to prevent scurvy. This alone makes it a worthwhile bit of information to have. It also has malic acid, calcium malate, dihydrofisetin, fisetin, iodine, gallic acid, tannic acid, selenium, and tartaric acid.

It has long been used as a folk medicine and has been the subject of research in modern medicine.

As far as a recipe—it's pretty much all to taste and pretty simple.

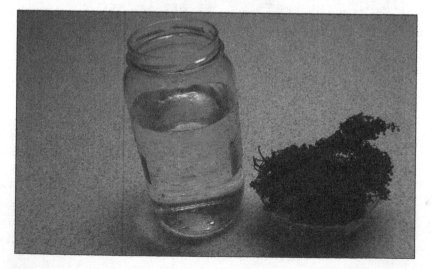

INGREDIENTS:

- Sumac berries
- Water
- Sugar (to taste)

PREPARATION

- Pick the sumac around August in order to make sure it is ripe.
- Don't pick the sumac cones after rain since the flavor comes from the sap on the outside of the berries.
- Remove as many leaves and twigs as possible. The more stems, the more tannic acid you will get.
- Place the sumac berries in a container filled with fresh cold water. You'll want about 1 cup of water for each cone. Warm water will make your drink bitter.
- Crush the berries with your hands.
- Let rest for about 30–60 minutes depending on how strong of a flavor you want.
- Strain using cheesecloth and sweeten to your liking. Serve cold with ice.

Personally, while I have to have sugar in my tea, I don't feel that sumac-ade needs sweeteners.

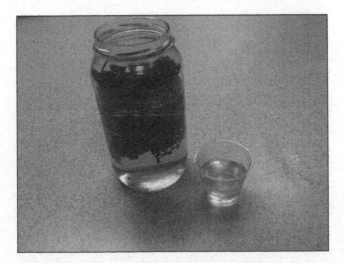

CHAPTER 17

PROJECT: HOW TO EAT ACORNS

Acorns have been tested and found to be one of the best foods for effectively controlling blood sugar levels. They have low sugar content, but leave a sweetish aftertaste, making them very good in stews, as well as in breads of all types.

The only two problems I have with eating acorns are that I am too lazy to pick them up quickly enough to prevent worms from ruining them, and that the tannins give them a bitter taste. Luckily there are solutions to both problems, and this project will teach you them.

This year I decided to harvest acorns from the oak trees in my front yard. Being lazy, I spread out a large tarp and weighted it down with rocks. Every afternoon (or so) from September to early November I would take a quick look and scoop up any acorns I saw on the tarp. If the acorns were soft feeling or looked like they were compromised, I tossed them down the hill; the good ones went inside with me to collect in a place where they would not be subject to rot or worms.

Once I got enough acorns to make the process worthwhile I processed them to remove the tannins. Tannic acid makes the acorns bitter, but different oak trees have differing amounts of tannins in the acorns. Depending on the oak tree and your taste buds, it may be possible to eat the acorns without any processing.

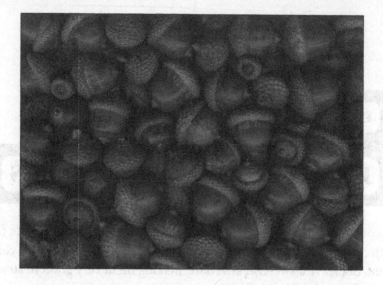

Unfortunately, oaks with that low of a tannin level are rare (Native Americans fought wars over them). They are also normally found on the West Coast. Beware that eating acorns without removing the tannins will make your mouth feel like cotton, can cause constipation, and, with large amounts, can even cause kidney damage. Luckily, to process your acorns all you really need is water.

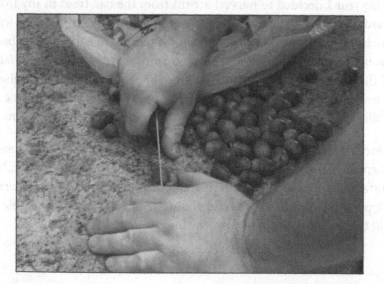

Native Americans basically threw their acorns in baskets and left them in swiftly running streams until the tannins were leeched out. For us modern folks, there are faster ways.

First thing to do is dry them out so that they don't mold. You can lay them out on a sheet or tarp, single layer deep, and let the sun cook them. Personally, I would rather throw them in the dehydrator for a couple hours, or put them on a cookie sheet in the oven at its lowest temperature (about 175°F) for about an hour.

Next, peel the acorn; it's simple to crack the shell with a nutcracker or slip joint pliers, peel off the thin skin, and throw the good acorns in a bucket. If the acorn has a black hole it is evidence of worm infestation—throw those out.

Next, get your food grinder and make a course meal. Put the meal in a pot and cover with boiling water. After an hour the water should be brown to black. You can throw this out; however, I have heard of using the tannin water to tan animal hides. Taste the meal: if it tastes sweet, it's done; if it's like eating a green persimmon, repeat the boiling water soak. Do this as many times as necessary.

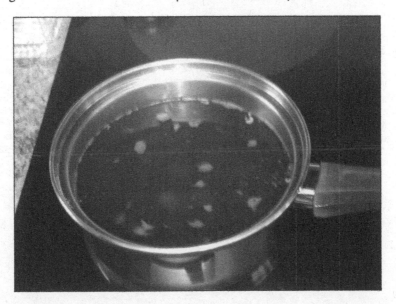

Once you are happy with the meal, lay it out to dry. A good way to start this process is to dump the wet meal in a sheet or doubled sheet of cheesecloth, gather the ends like a jelly bag, and press the water out. Next, put it in the oven at its lowest setting or in a dehydrator. Be careful with this process, as if you let the meal sit around wet it will mold.

In an airtight jar the coarsely ground chunks will last a while in the freezer. Grind it to flour as you need it, because the acorn oil will go rancid about as fast as whole grains will. Either way, course or fine, it will start go rancid in a couple weeks if stored at room temperature.

You can use acorn meal in many of the same ways as wheat flour. I have seen recipes online for acorn pasta, pancakes, and various breads.

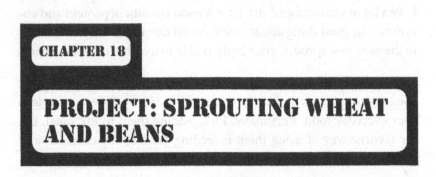

CHAPTER 18

PROJECT: SPROUTING WHEAT AND BEANS

We all know that nothing is free, especially food storage. Finding foods that are cost effective and long storing generally means you have less of the two vs—variety and vitamins. Sprouting is a way to add both. I used to associate sprouts with homeopathic medicine practitioners, vegans, and yuppie soccer moms, but once I got over my initial prejudice I learned that it's simple and cheap to add sprouts to my food toolbox.

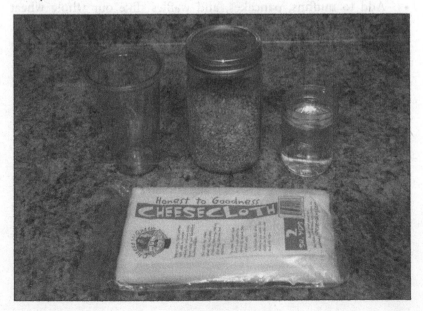

Studies show that sprouts have 3 to 5 times the vitamin content of the seed they sprouted from. And as for vitamins, sprouts have over 30 times the vitamin C content of the original seed. Wheat grain sprouts have a lot of vitamins and also have a good amount of protein and enzymes. The great thing about wheat is that due to the enzyme actions in the seed as it sprouts, your body is able to use the nutrients inside.

There are all sorts of recipes online for sprouts, and I would suggest you try a couple now and see how easy it is to incorporate sprouts into your everyday food. Personally, I like adding them to my salad, but my favorite way of using them is feeding them to my chickens and eating the eggs they produce. . . .

HOW TO USE SPROUTED WHEAT:
- Add either chopped or whole to homemade bread
- Add to oatmeal or other whole grain cereal
- Stir into cooked rice
- Add to rice pilaf
- Knead into pizza dough
- Chop and add to cookies
- Add to muffins, pancakes, and waffles (like our whole wheat pancakes)
- Add to casseroles, stuffed peppers, meatloaf, meatballs, pasta sauce, and mushroom sauces
- Add to sandwiches
- Sprinkle on yogurt
- Sprinkle in salads
- In stir fry

EQUIPMENT:
- Wide-mouthed jar (or something similar)
- Nylon net or cheesecloth and rubber band (to cover the jar and keep the cover in place)

INGREDIENTS:
- ½ cup wheat berries
- Water

PROCEDURE:

- Rinse ½ cup of wheat berries.
- Put the wheat berries in a wide-mouth quart jar.
- Add 2 cups of room temperature water.
- Place nylon net or cheesecloth over the jar opening.

> Don't put too many berries in the jar—no more than ½ cup per wide-mouth jar.

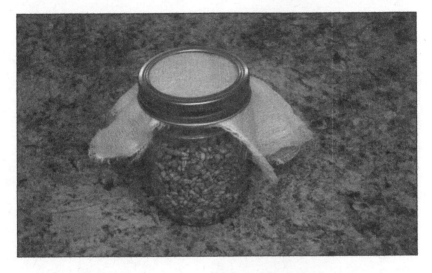

- Use a heavy rubber band or the metal jar ring to hold the nylon or cheesecloth in place.
- Soak 12 hours, then drain.
- Thoroughly drain the water—shake a bit to remove most of the water.
- Keep the jar out of direct sunlight.
- It needs the air, so keep cheesecloth as a lid.
- Each morning and night rinse the wheat berries with room temperature water, drain again. Taste after each soaking, Some keep the liquid drained off and drink it; I have done this, but I don't like the taste—even if I did feel a burst of energy after drinking it.
- 36 to 48 hours after the first soaking, voila! You have germinated wheat, and if you continue the process for a day or two more you will have sprouted wheat.

STORING WHEAT SPROUTS:

Replace the nylon net or cheesecloth with plastic wrap or the metal jar lid to help keep it moist but not wet. Store in cool place for no more than 5 days.

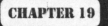

CHAPTER 19

HYGIENE IN THE FIELD

In a survival situation, cleanliness is essential to prevent infection. Adequate personal cleanliness will not only protect against disease germs that are present in the individual's surroundings, but will also protect the group by reducing the spread of these germs.

a. Washing, particularly the face, hands, and feet, reduces the chances of infection from small scratches and abrasions. A daily bath or shower with hot water and soap is ideal. If no tub or shower is available, the body should be cleaned with a cloth and soapy water, paying particular attention to the body creases (armpits, groin, etc.), face, ears, hands, and feet. After this type of "bath," the body should be rinsed thoroughly with clear water to remove all traces of soap which could cause irritation.

b. Soap, although an aid, is not essential to keeping clean. Ashes, sand, loamy soil, and other expedients may be used to clean the body and cooking utensils.

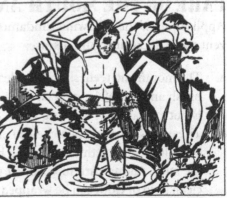

c. When water is in short supply, the survivor should take an "air bath." All clothing should be removed and the body simply exposed to the air. Exposure to sunshine is ideal, but even on an overcast day or indoors, a 2-hour exposure of the naked body to the air will refresh the body. Care should be taken to avoid sunburn when bathing in this manner. Exposure in the shade, shelter, sleeping bag, etc., will help if the weather conditions do not permit direct exposure.

d. Hair should be kept trimmed, preferably 2 inches or less in length, and the face should be clean-shaven. Hair provides a surface for the attachment of parasites and the growth of bacteria. Keeping the hair short and the face clean-shaven will provide less habitat for these organisms. At least once a week, the hair should be washed with soap and water. When water is in short supply, the hair should be combed or brushed thoroughly and covered to keep it clean. It should be inspected weekly for fleas, lice, and other parasites. When parasites are discovered, they should be removed.

e. The principal means of infecting food and open wounds is contact with unclean hands. Hands should be washed with soap and water, if available, after handling any material which is likely to carry germs. This is especially important after each visit to the latrine, when caring for the sick and injured, and before handling food, food utensils, or drinking water. The fingers should be kept out of the mouth and the fingernails kept closely trimmed and clean. A scratch from a long fingernail could develop into a serious infection.

CARE OF THE MOUTH AND TEETH

Application of the following fundamentals of oral hygiene will prevent tooth decay and gum disease:

a. The mouth and teeth should be cleansed thoroughly with a toothbrush and dentifrice at least once each day. When a toothbrush is not available, a "chewing stick" can be fashioned from a twig. The twig is washed, then chewed on one end until it is frayed and brushlike. The teeth can then be brushed very thoroughly with the stick, taking care to clean all tooth surfaces. If necessary, a clean strip of cloth can be wrapped around the finger and rubbed on the teeth to wipe away food particles which have collected on them. When neither toothpaste nor toothpowder are available, salt, soap, or baking soda can be used as substitute dentifrices. Parachute inner core can be used by separating the filaments of the inner core and using this as a dental floss. Gargling with willow bark tea will help protect the teeth.

b. Food debris which has accumulated between the teeth should be removed by using dental floss or toothpicks. The latter can be fashioned from small twigs.

c. Gum tissues should be stimulated by rubbing them vigorously with a clean finger each day.

d. Use as much care cleaning dentures and other dental applianc-es, removable or fixed, as when cleaning natural teeth. Dentures and removable bridges should be removed and cleaned with a denture brush or "chew stick" at least once each day. The tissue under the dentures should be brushed or rubbed regularly for proper stimulation. Removable dental appliances should be re-moved at night or for a 2 to 3-hour period during the day.

CARE OF THE FEET

Proper care of the feet is of utmost importance in a survival situation, especially if the survivor has to travel. Serious foot trouble can be prevented by observing the fol-lowing simple rules:

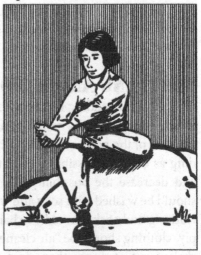

a. The feet should be washed, dried thoroughly, and mas-saged each day. If water is in short supply, the feet should be "air cleaned" along with the rest of the body.

b. Toenails should be trimmed straight across to prevent the development of ingrown toenails.

Care of the feet.

c. Boots should be broken in before wearing them on any mission. They should fit properly, neither so tight that they bind and cause pressure spots nor so loose that they permit the foot to slide forward and backward when walking. Insoles should be improvised to reduce any friction spots inside the shoes.

d. Socks should be large enough to allow the toes to move freely but not so loose that they wrinkle. Wool socks should be at least one size larger than cotton socks to allow for shrinkage. Socks with holes should be properly darned before they are worn. Wearing socks with holes or socks that are poorly repaired may cause blisters. Clots of wool on the inside and outside should be removed from wool socks because they may cause blisters. Socks should be changed and washed thoroughly with soap and water each day. Woolen socks should be washed in cool water to lessen shrinkage. In camp, freshly laundered socks should be stretched to facilitate drying by hanging in the sun or in an air current. While traveling, a damp pair of socks can be dried by placing them inside layers of clothing or hanging them on the outside of the pack. If socks become damp, they should be exchanged for dry ones at the first opportunity.

e. When traveling, the feet should be examined regularly to see if there are any red spots or blisters. If detected in the early stages of development, tender areas should be covered with adhesive tape to prevent blister formation.

CLOTHING AND BEDDING

Clothing and bedding become contaminated with any disease germs which may be present on the skin, in the stool, in the urine, or in secretions of the nose and throat. Therefore, keeping clothing and bedding as clean as possible will decrease the chances of skin infection and decrease the possibility of parasite infestation. Outer clothing should be washed with soap and water when it becomes soiled. Under clothing and socks should be changed daily. If water is in short supply, clothing should be "air cleaned." For air cleaning, the clothing is shaken out of doors, then aired and sunned for 2 hours. Clothing cleaned in this manner should be worn in rotation. Sleeping bags should be turned inside out, fluffed, and aired after each use. Bed linen should be changed at least once a week, and the blankets, pillows, and mattresses should be aired and sunned.

REST

Rest is necessary for the survivor because it not only restores physical and mental vigor, but also promotes healing during an illness or after an injury.

a. In the initial stage of the survival episode, rest is particularly important. After those tasks requiring immediate attention are done, the survivor should inventory available resources, decide upon a plan of action, and even have a meal. This "planning session" will provide a rest period without the survivor having a feeling of "doing nothing."

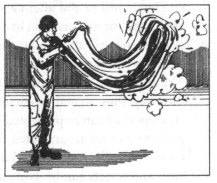
Bedding.

b. If possible, regular rest periods should be planned in each day's activities. The amount of time allotted for rest will depend on a number of factors, including the survivor's physical condition, the presence of hostile forces, etc., but usually, 10 minutes each hour is sufficient. During these rest periods, the survivor should change either from physical activity to complete rest or from mental activity to physical activity as the case may be. The survivor must learn to become comfortable and to rest under less than ideal conditions.'

RULES FOR AVOIDING ILLNESS

In a survival situation, whether short-term or long-term, the dangers of disease are multiplied. Application of the following simple guidelines regarding personal hygiene will enable the survivor to safeguard personal health and the health of others:

a. ALL water obtained from natural sources should be purified before consumption.

b. The ground in the camp area should not be soiled with urine or feces. Latrines should be used, if available. When no latrines are available, individuals should dig "cat holes" and cover their waste.

c. Fingers and other contaminated objects should never be put into the mouth. Hands should be washed before handling any food or drinking water, before using the fingers in the care of the mouth and teeth, before and after caring for the sick and injured, and after handling any material likely to carry disease germs.

d. After each meal, all eating utensils should be cleaned and disinfected in boiling water.

e. The mouth and teeth should be cleansed thoroughly at least once each day. Most dental problems associated with long-term survival episodes can be prevented by using a toothbrush and toothpaste to remove accumulated food debris. If necessary, devices for cleaning the teeth should be improvised.

f. Bites and insects can be avoided by keeping the body clean, by wearing proper protective clothing, and by using head nets, improvised bed nets, and insect repellants.

g. Wet clothing should be exchanged for dry clothing as soon as possible to avoid unnecessary body heat loss.

h. Personal items such as canteens, pipes, towels, toothbrushes, handkerchiefs, and shaving items should not be shared with others.

i. All food scraps, cans, and refuse should be removed from the camp area and buried.

j. If possible, a survivor should get 7 or 8 hours of sleep each night.

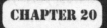

CHAPTER 20

BOOTS AND FOOT CARE

For many of us who hunt, hike or do a lot of walking in the outdoors, some of the most overlooked pieces of equipment center around our feet. At the same time, there are others who are quite serious about hiking and acquire quality equipment by purchasing the right socks, hiking or hunting boots and who appropriately take care of them. In a state like Pennsylvania, where over a million hunting licenses are sold each year, that single outdoor activity translates into over a million individuals trekking around out there in all kinds of weather. It is obvious that some of those million individuals will end up with sore feet after that first day outdoors. Due to sore or blistered feet, there is not a second day or if there is, it is a painful one. Unfortunately many people purchase the right footwear but still end-up with blisters. To avoid these pitfalls, precautions must be taken.

To get advice on this, I asked two individuals in the footwear industry for some of their ideas on foot care and safety. For hunting boots, I spoke with Krystal Krage from Irish Setter Inc. Here are some of her ideas on outdoor boots. Hunting boots can be divided into different categories based on terrain and weather conditions that you expect to encounter. The upper materials, linings, soles and construction are the variables that make these boots perform properly in different environments.

The two primary types of hunting boots are upland boots and big game boots. To properly select a boot, consider what conditions and terrain you'll be walking through, the wetness of the environment, the temperature and the general conditions underfoot.

BOOTS IN GENERAL

The upper is the part of the boot that's above the sole. It supports your ankle and protects your foot. Upper materials are usually leather, or leather combined with tough nylon fabric. Leather provides excellent support and protection and will be sturdier than most fabrics in rocky conditions. Fabric panels, on the other hand, can make the boot more lightweight and flexible. Leather quality can vary quite a bit as well. The top of the line is full-grain waterproof or water resistant leather. Lower-priced boots often incorporate more nylon or use split leathers.

The gusset is the part of the boot where the tongue meets the rest of the boot. This area may be padded for extra comfort when you pull the laces tight to get a secure fit. When you look for a boot, choose one that fits snugly and comfortably so there's less movement of your foot in the boot. Movement within the boot is what leads to "hot spots" or blisters that can make the day seem very long. Pay particular attention to how the widest part of the foot fits in the widest part of the boot and make sure you have the proper width so that toes are not cramped. If you are high-arched or flat-footed, look for boots with addable insoles that allow for more of a custom fit.

BOOT HEIGHT

Boots come in various heights that offer differ ent levels of support. These can range form 7-inch hiker styles to 18-inch snake boots. When selecting a pair of boots, pay attention to where the top of the collar meets your leg. You want a boot that will minimize rubbing! Also feel the padding on the collar and select what feels the best to you. Try on a few different pairs before making a purchase to see which style fits your foot and leg best.

WATERPROOFING

Waterproofing is extremely important. If you're in the back country with cold, wet feet, it can lead to a medical emergency. If you will be walking through dewy grass in the morning, you may only need water-resistant leather without a waterproofing system. Gore-Tex material is a well known waterproof and breathable waterproofing system used in much outdoor equipment.

INSULATION

Insulation is a major consideration in footwear selection. If you're planning to hunt in a warm climate, you'll probably want non-insulated footwear. For cold weather, an insulated boot is desirable. Many boot manufacturers use Thinsulate or Thermolite insulation which is measured in grams. For example, two hundred grams is the least amount of insulation you can buy. Insulation numbers increase from there to 1600 grams. When purchasing a hunting boot, choose your insulation need by the air temperature, ground temperature and the amount of foot movement you anticipate. You'll need to balance your need for a non-sweaty walk with your need for a comfortably warm foot when you're stationary.

SOLES

These provide varying levels of traction, cushioning, shock absorption, lateral stability and flexibility. They can be incredibly lightweight and not very durable but you wouldn't want to walk very far in such a boot. Most hiking, backpacking and hunting boots use soles that are somewhere in between. Tread size is also critical when selecting a boot. A shallow tread works best for varying upland terrain where you want to limit the amount of mud and debris that the treads pick up. An aggressive tread with an air bob design works best for mountainous and hilly terrain.

SNAKEPROOFING

Since hunters, fishermen and hikers get into areas where there are venomous snakes, leg protection is a concern. What makes a boot snake-proof? The best protection comes from tightly woven 1,000 denier basket weave nylon uppers and a snake guard backer. A thorn guard backer is lined through the entire boot for added durability and simply put, the snake guard backer is just a beefed-up version of the thorn guard. From reports by those who have been struck by poisonous snakes, these boots have been field tested and they prevented individuals from being bitten. A person struck by a snake while wearing these boots might be a bit shaken, but will not have his skin penetrated by the fangs and will walk away unharmed. If you are going to be in such areas, such protection is simply common sense insurance.

CORDURA VERSUS LEATHER

Another factor to consider when choosing boots is the material from which they are made. Cordura nylon boots have been a hit with hunters and hikers across the country since this material is light-weight and requires little maintenance. Once a Cordura boot gets muddy, simply wash it down with a soft brush and water and when dry, apply a silicon spray to help retain the boots water repellence. On the other hand, when it comes to all leather boots, although heavier, they provide a bit more support and rigidity when in extremely rugged terrain. Also, caring for a leather boot takes a bit more time and treating leather with a conditioner will extend the life of the boot. Then after treating, apply a silicon spray which will help the leather repel water. Basically, no matter what you elect to purchase, you must care for the boot as suggested by the manufacturer and when needed, apply a conditioner and water repellent to assure that your footwear will serve you for many years.

COMMON FOOTWEAR MYTHS

"If I buy good hunting boots, I don't have to break them in." Not true! The best boots need breaking in. Boots need to conform to your feet, and your feet have to get used to the boots. The sturdiest boots require the longest breaking in, but end up being the most comfortable. Here's another great tip for your feet: get them in shape before the hunting season, not during the hunting season. Get started by walking and constantly increase the distance until you are not out of breadth and your feet feel good in the boot you will be using for hunting. This will put both your feet and body in shape before the season begins.

"If your feet are cold, add more socks." The truth of the matter is, the number of socks you wear has little to do with overall foot warmth.

As a matter of fact, the more socks you jam into your boots, the colder your feet will be. Your feet need room to breathe and the better they breathe, the warmer they'll be. The tighter your boots, the faster your feet will get cold since circulation will also be hampered.

SOME RULES TO CONSIDER ABOUT BOOTS & SOCKS

- Buy new boots with the socks you plan to wear outdoors to get a proper fit.
- Always wear proper socks.
- Wear a thin liner (polypropylene or Thermax) next to your feet to wick moisture away.
- Next, wear a wool sock! Wool's hollow-core fiber will further wick moisture away from your feet which keeps them dry and warm.

Socks & Boots as Medical Concerns Before putting on your boots, consider socks. Be careful with designs that have heavy gummed tops meant to hold up your socks. When this is too tight, circulation can be cut when moving, especially in cold weather. You need good blood circulation and don't want to be hampered by the tops of tight socks that turn into a light tourniquet.

SPECIAL CONCERNS FOR DIABETICS–A good pair of shoes or boots can be a healthy choice for everyone but can be a "must" for a few. A major medical concern for those who have diabetes mel litus is the feet, since these individuals are at special risk for foot problems. With diabetes there can be a deterioration of blood vessels and nerves in the hands and feet. This can then limit blood flow to these areas which may lead to gangrene.

If you are a diabetic, be aware of complications to your feet which can manifest as circulatory problems, diabetic neuropathy (along with a decrease in circulation, one may also experience a loss of sensitivity and nerve loss in the feet which due to numbing, affects one's ability to experience pain which can be a warning that something like a blister is forming) and foot infections.

Proper foot care along with proper socks and boot fit is critical for these individuals. It is a good idea for anyone, but especially for diabetics, to examine their feet for any friction rubs and make sure their socks are not bunched and that their footwear fits properly, allowing for unobstructed circulation.

BLISTERS–These are collections of clear fluid that accumulate in a specific area under the skin. The result is a raised section of skin that is now quite tender and sore. A blister is caused by constant rubbing of an area from a shoe that does not properly fit. Large blisters, more than a half-inch in diameter, are medically referred to as bullae. A smaller raised area or blister is referred to as a vesicle. The resulting damage under these rubs are "abused" small blood vessels within the traumatized area. Now what happens is the leaking of serum from these traumatized blood vessels, and the formation of a blister.

The serum is usually sterile and therefore, if the skin of the blister is not broken, the blister provides protection to the area that was damaged by the friction.

By knowing that friction is the enemy that causes a blister, it should be a little easier to prevent them through sensible countermeasures. What first happens in this chain of events is that, as you are walking, friction on an area causes a "hot spot" or "thermal burn." When this happens it soon becomes uncomfortable — this is your body putting out a warning for you to take action or pay later. Again, by understanding that friction is the cause, it becomes evident that further rubbing of that area must be halted. To do this, take off your shoe and sock and cover the area in question with something like smooth surface tape or mole skin.

Remember that the skin on your feet is smooth when dry but becomes tender when hot and wet from perspiration. It is a good idea to carry a second pair of socks so that, if the first pair becomes wet or damp, you can change into a dry pair.

When you put your sock back on, make sure there are no creases in it since this will act like a foreign body in your shoe. Also, inspect and empty out your boot to make sure that there are no irritating objects, such as a pebble or splinter. If you develop a blister and have to keep walking, a controlled break may be your best bet to reduce discomfort and lessen the chance of more tissue damage if it breaks on its own. Once blisters form, the serum under the skin adds pressure which is quite uncomfortable. You can open and drain the blister using a sterile needle (sterilize the needle by holding it in an open flame), and then cover it with a sterile dressing for a day or two.

Unfortunately, with this treatment you have caused another potential problem. Because the blister was a closed area and the serum was likely sterile, it has now been opened and drained and bacteria can get in through the drainage hole. Emergency First Aid for a Blister

- Apply a smooth dressing and adjust socks to prevent further irritation.

IF YOU NEED TO DRAIN A BLISTER
- Wash the blistered area with soap and clean water and wipe it with an alcohol swab.
- Drain the blister by making a small opening at the edge using a sterile needle or knife tip.
- Keep the blistered area clean and covered with a sterile dressing.

MOLESKIN BLISTER CUSHION
For another approach to blister first aid, you can build a cushion with layers of moleskin in which holes have been cut to accommodate the intact blister. If you are worried about infection, or are a diabetic, this may be the best approach. To play it safe, always contact your family physician or podiatrist when you can for their recommendations. Especially if you are a diabetic, you need to contact your health care provider who knows your situation and therefore can best adjust the treatment to your particular circumstances.

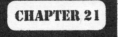

CHAPTER 21

WILDERNESS FIRST-AID

COLD INJURY/FROSTBITE

GENERAL COMMENTS
Cold exposure can cause both freezing and non-freezing injuries—depending on the depth of the skin layers involved. Frostnip leads to numb, pale, soft skin whereas frostbite is the actual freezing of cells and a more severe cold injury. Cold injuries range from minor pain to extreme pain on rewarming and often permanent disability. Extremities are most prone to cold injury (ear lobes, nose, fingers, and toes). Factors contributing to cold injury include: hypothermia, prior frostbite, dehydration, constricting clothing/ boots, wind, severity of cold environment, wetness, and concurrent alcohol or tobacco use. Rewarm/thaw the involved extremity as soon as possible to decrease eventual tissue damage, unless there is a chance of refreezing. Refreezing of the thawed extremity will worsen outcomes and the viability of affected tissue. It may be better to walk the patient out on frozen feet than to risk thawing and then refreezing the injury.

SYMPTOMS
- Pale, white, waxy, hard skin, numbness (may feel like a "chunk of wood").
- Blanching of extremities (pinking of nail bed after pressure takes > 3 seconds).
- Blisters (clear).

- Mottled, dusky, "bluish" skin.
- After rewarming: Skin is swollen, red, painful.
- May develop clear blisters
- May develop blood-filled blisters (represents a deep tissue injury).
- **Red Flags:** Dusky mottled skin, blood-filled blisters.

TREATMENT:

- Primary treatment is the rapid rewarming of frozen extremity only if there is no risk of refreezing.
- Thaw with non-scalding water (104°F–106°F), should be hot-tub temperature.
- Keep affected extremity submerged for 20–30 minutes or until skin becomes soft and returns to normal color (may need to re-heat water).
- Ibuprofen or Tylenol as needed for pain.
- Dress with gauze between fingers or toes and around extremity.
- Do not rewarm with radiant heat (fire).
- Do not massage or rub with snow.
- Blisters: drain clear blisters (see Blisters); do not drain blood-filled blisters.

EVACUATE:

- Any patient with blood-filled blisters
- Dusky, blotchy, skin.
- If unable to use the injured extremity due to either pain or immobility.
- If unable to protect area from further cold or refreezing.
- Any patient whose pain cannot be managed in the field.
- Any signs of infection to affected area.

HEAT ILLNESS

GENERAL COMMENTS

Heat-related illnesses might be due to overexertion, under-or ove-rhydration, or medications that exacerbate the body's response to a hot environment. An accurate patient history may be more helpful than a thermometer. Overhydration with plain water while excessively sweating may lead to a dangerous depletion of the body's salt balance. Always rehydrate with electrolyte containing fluids and/or salty foods. Exertion in hot climates may expose one to heat exhaustion or heat stroke. A person is more susceptible to heat illness while on certain medications (some cardiac medicines, high blood pressure medicines, anti-anxiety/depressants, over-the-counter cold medicines, alcohol, stimulants) or in humid conditions. Cold water immersion is the best way to rapidly cool someone with heat illness—immerse up to level of nipples and be cautious to keep shoulders and head dry and secure in case of loss of consciousness.

SYMPTOMS: LOW SALT LEVEL (HYPONATREMIA)
- Weakness, nausea, dizziness, or muscle cramps.
- Altered LOR (without elevated temperature).
- Seizures.
- **Red flag:** Altered LOR, seizures.

TREATMENT:
- Rehydrate with dilute solution of sugar drink with salt or with an electrolyte solution.
- Provide gradual intake of salty foods.

SYMPTOMS: HEAT EXHAUSTION
- Flushed, rapid pulse, sweating, dizzy, nausea, headache, chills, history of decreased water intake and/or decreased urine output.
- Crampy abdominal pain.
- **Red flags:** Dark yellow or bloody urine, decreased urine output, predisposing medications.

TREATMENT:
- Stop exertion and rest in shade.
- Rehydrate with electrolyte containing fluids.
- Gentle stretching for cramps.
- Evaporative cooling: Wet the victim's clothes/head and make a fan/draft to dissipate heat through evaporation.
- Cool with wet cloth.

SYMPTOMS: HEAT STROKE
- Symptoms of heat exhaustion but with altered LOR
- Seizures
- Patient may be sweating or have dry skin, may be flushed or pale.

TREATMENT:
- Similar treatment for heat exhaustion with aggressive cooling: Cold water immersion is first choice (if available), otherwise, evaporative cooling.
- Cautious hydration of the patient with altered LOR, as they are at risk of seizures and subsequent vomiting and aspiration.

EVACUATE:
- Heat stroke (or any altered LOR)—these should have EMS brought to them to minimize exertion and further heat generation.
- Persistent symptoms of heat exhaustion that do not improve.
- Red/brown urine.

HYPOTHERMIA

GENERAL COMMENTS
Hypothermia occurs when the body's ability to produce and retain heat is overwhelmed by the cold effect. Wind and moisture lead to more rapid and severe heat loss. Hypothermia treatment has three main focuses: (1) minimize the effect of cold, (2) increase heat production, and (3) minimize heat loss.

The clinical presentation of hypothermia is more important than the patient's temperature, as it may be difficult to obtain an accurate temperature in the field. Mild hypothermia can effectively be managed, but any symptoms of severe hypothermia must be recognized early, as the wilderness setting offers limited reheating methods. The rescuer may be limited to minimizing cold effect and heat loss. Recognize that severe hypothermia will likely require evacuation and rewarming via EMS.

SYMPTOMS: MILD HYPOTHERMIA (90–95°F)

- Shivering (persistent).
- Loss of fine motor coordination (stumbling).
- Withdrawn or irritable, confusion, and/or poor judgment.

TREATMENT:

- Change the environment and find shelter.
- Replace wet clothing with dry clothing, add wind and waterproof layers.
- Add insulation under and around the patient.
- Cover head and neck.
- Hot/sweet liquids and food (calories).

SYMPTOMS: SEVERE HYPOTHERMIA (< 90°F)

- Cessation of shivering (at 86°F).
- Altered LOR, lethargic and may seem drunk.
- Combative or irrational.
- Slowed heart rate and respiratory rate.
- May appear in coma.

TREATMENT:

- Evacuate, as unlikely able to increase core temperature.
- Minimize heat loss and cold exposure. Wrap in sleeping bag with a warm hat.
- If altered LOR, be cautious giving fluids or food because of the risk of vomiting and aspiration.
- If in a coma, handle patient gently as heart is prone to fatal heart rhythms.
- Hypothermia wrap.

EVACUATE:

- Mild hypothermia that you are not able to rewarm.
- Severe hypothermia.

SKIN IRRITATION

GENERAL COMMENTS
Take care to educate yourself on identifying toxic plants, such as poison oak, poison ivy, stinging nettle, and poison sumac. Many skin irritations can be prevented though improved hygiene practices and appropriate clothing. The active ingredient that causes the reaction is oil that can be transferred to the skin. Inhaled smoke from burning plants can also cause a reaction.

SYMPTOMS
- Itchy red rash, fluid-filled blisters. Blisters may be delayed for several days.

TREATMENT:
- Rapidly wash the affected area (or suspected exposed area) well with soap and water.
- Wash all clothes and equipment that may have been exposed.
- Once the rash appears, itching can be relieved with of Hydrocortisone cream. More severe itching can be treated with Benadryl.

EVACUATE:
- Any reaction that involves the eyes, genitals, lips, mouth, or breathing.
- Skin irritation that is too uncomfortable to continue trip.
- Any signs of infection to skin (e.g., spreading redness, warmth, and/or pus).

TOXINS, BITES & STINGS

GENERAL COMMENTS
The effects of an irritating toxin can range from a mild local reaction to critical systemic involvement. The inciting agent may be difficult to identify. Regardless, the goals of treatment are the same: minimize exposure, dilute (if possible), and maximize excretion of the toxin.

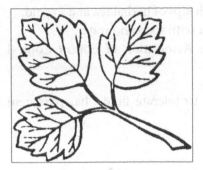

Poison oak.

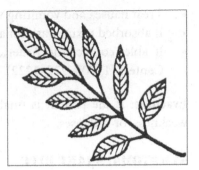

Poison sumac.

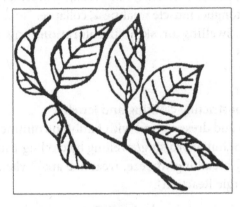

Poison ivy.

Give symptomatic support, as specific antidotes are unlikely to be available in the wilderness environment. Fatalities due to bites, stings, or other envenomations are rare and may be due to anaphylaxis (see Allergic Reaction). While most bites and stings do not lead to more than a local reaction (or none at all), symptoms can worsen and progress, so evacuate all snake bites or scorpion stings.

SYMPTOMS: INGESTED TOXIN

- Mild nausea, vomiting, diarrhea, headache, collapse, seizures.

TREATMENT:

- Remove patient from offending toxin (e.g., tent with stove possibly causing carbon monoxide toxicity).

- Treat nausea and vomiting with sips of herbal tea and Pepcid.
- If absorbed toxin, wash off area with soap and water.
- If able, contact the American Association of Poison Control Centers (1–800–222–1222).

Evacuate: If the patient is unable to tolerate fluids, has persistent weakness, or collapses.

SYMPTOMS: SNAKE BITE
- Oozing at site, significant pain from bite, swelling, bruising, discoloration, possible shortness of breath, wheezing, numbness to mouth or tongue, muscle weakness, collapse.
- **Red flag:** Swelling or skin discoloration, any neurological symptoms.

TREATMENT:
- Remove constricting clothing and jewelry.
- Clean area and dress wound with antibiotic ointment.
- Mark site of initial bruising/swelling by circling with a pen.
- If difficulty breathing/wheeze, treat like anaphylaxis (see Severe under Allergic Reaction).
- Evacuate.

Evacuate: All snake bites, regardless of swelling or bruising, as symptoms may progress over 6–8 hours. Ambulate if able, otherwise send for EMS.

SYMPTOMS: STINGS OR BITES (INSECTS, BEES, WASPS, ANTS, TICKS)
- Local pain, swelling, redness, weakness, nausea, vomiting, fever.
- Allergic reaction.

TREATMENT:
- Scrape off stinger.
- If tick is imbedded, grab the head with tweezers as near the skin as possible, and with constant gentle force pull up and away.

- Wash area well with soap and water.
- Cold compress to area.
- Benadryl for local inflammation/itching (see Allergic Reaction).
- If difficulty breathing/wheeze, treat like anaphylaxis (see Severe under Allergic Reaction).

Evacuate: Any sting with associated breathing difficulties or severe allergic reaction/anaphylaxis.

SYMPTOMS: SPIDER BITE
- Pin prick or painless bite, severe muscle cramps and pain in bitten extremity, may involve stomach or chest muscles, blistering or redness to site.

TREATMENT:
- Clean bite with soap and water.
- Ibuprofen or Tylenol as needed for pain.
- Cold compress to area.

Evacuate: If severe pain within 60 minutes of bite.

SYMPTOMS: SCORPION STING
- Painful sting, burning pain to site, numbness to site, paralysis, muscle spasms, blurred vision, swallowing difficulty, breathing problems, slurred speech.

TREATMENT:
- Cool compress to site.
- Ibuprofen or Tylenol as needed for pain.

Evacuate: All scorpion stings. Symptoms may progress over 6–8 hours, evacuate early.

SYMPTOMS: JELLYFISH
- Skin irritation, severe burning, itching, nausea and vomiting, headache, muscle aches, dizziness, numbness, seizure, collapse, altered LOR.

TREATMENT:
- Rinse wound with seawater (avoid freshwater).
- Rinse with vinegar (avoid vinegar if suspected Man O' War).
- Make a paste of sand and water; scrape off extra stinging cells with edge of card/knife.
- Apply hot water after stinging cells have been scraped off.
- If allergic reaction or anaphylaxis, treat accordingly.

Evacuate: Severe pain, any severe allergic reaction, or any breathing problems or neurological problems.

NOTES

NOTES

NOTES

NOTES

NOTES

NOTES

NOTES